FUNDAMENTALS of GASTROINTESTINAL RADIOLOGY

Michael Davis, M.D.
Professor Emeritus of Radiology
Past Chief of Gastrointestinal and
    Genitourinary Radiology
Department of Radiology
University of New Mexico
    Health Sciences Center
Albuquerque, New Mexico

Jeffrey D. Houston, M.D.
Department of Radiology
University of New Mexico
    Health Sciences Center
Albuquerque, New Mexico

D1477224

W.B. SAUNDERS COMPANY
A Harcourt Health Sciences Company
Philadelphia   London   New York   St. Louis   Sydney   Toronto

W.B. SAUNDERS COMPANY
A Harcourt Health Sciences Company

The Curtis Center
Independence Square West
Philadelphia, Pennsylvania 19106

Library of Congress Cataloging-in-Publication Data

Fundamentals of gastrointestinal radiology / Michael Davis, Jeffrey D. Houston.—1st ed.

p.   cm.

Includes index.

ISBN 0–7216–5203–4

1. Gastrointestinal system—Radiography.   I. Davis, Michael
II. Houston, Jeffrey D.   III. Title.
[DNLM: 1. Gastrointestinal System—radiography.   WI 141 D263f 2002]

RC804.R6 D38 2002   616.3′307572—dc21

2001031369

Editor-in-Chief: Richard Lampert
Acquisitions Editor: Lisette Bralow
Developmental Editor: Gwen Wright
Illustration Specialist: Peg Shaw
Book Designer: Steven Stave

FUNDAMENTALS OF GASTROINTESTINAL RADIOLOGY   ISBN 0–7216–5203–4

Printed in the United States of America.

Last digit is the print number: 9   8   7   6   5   4   3   2   1

To Gae
MD

To Ken, for inspiring my pursuit of radiology
To Mick, for sharing his passion for GI radiology
To my family, for everything else
JDH

Contributors

CECILIA M. COUTSIAS, M.D.
Clinical Diagnostic Radiology
Phoenix, Arizona

DANICA C. HOLT, M.D.
San Gabriel Valley Diagnostic Center
West Covina, California

JULIE A. LOCKEN, M.D.
Assistant Professor of Radiology
Chief of Abdominal Imaging
Department of Radiology
University of New Mexico
Health Sciences Center
Albuquerque, New Mexico

Preface

The purpose of *Fundamentals of Gastrointestinal Radiology* is to provide an introduction to gastrointestinal radiology for medical students, residents, and other physicians who study or manage disorders of the gastrointestinal system. We strive not to provide a comprehensive reference text of the radiologic manifestations of gastrointestinal pathology, but to confer a concise overview of commonly encountered and radiologically unique disease entities. Representative images are provided to illustrate both normal and abnormal imaging findings.

The foundation for understanding abnormal radiologic images rests on a thorough knowledge of normal anatomy and its appearance, using various imaging modalities. We begin the discussion of each segment of the gastrointestinal system with an overview of the relevant anatomy, imaging techniques, and indications for examination. Perhaps the most important concept that we hope to impart to our readers is an understanding of which imaging examinations are indicated to optimally evaluate specific disease processes. It is of paramount importance for referring clinicians to understand the benefits and limitations of the various imaging examinations available to evaluate the gastrointestinal tract. The ability of the radiologist to diagnose disease is directly related to the appropriateness of the requested examination and the communication of the relevant clinical data. As the essence of radiology is the interpretation of images, our goal is to provide an appropriate amount of images for readers to become familiar with the essential radiologic abnormalities seen in the gastrointestinal tract.

As this book provides on overview of widely known concepts, we believe that it is unnecessary to provide specific references. Instead, we include lists of recommended readings at the conclusion of each chapter for those readers who wish to explore specific topics in further detail. We hope that this book provides a practical and concise introduction to gastrointestinal radiology.

Michael Davis, M.D.
Jeffrey D. Houston, M.D.

Acknowledgments

We wish to acknowledge our colleagues, the radiology technologists, and the support personnel from the Department of Radiology at the University of New Mexico Health Sciences Center for providing the material for this book. We especially thank Charlotte A. Hendrix for her valuable editorial assistance and perseverance in assembling our long overdue manuscript. Likewise, we thank Joseph C. Tafoya, whose photographic expertise has been invaluable in the completion of this book.

Contents

ONE

Introduction to Gastrointestinal Radiology

Jeffrey D. Houston, M.D., and Michael Davis, M.D.

Gastrointestinal radiology encompasses the radiologic imaging of a wide variety of functional and structural abnormalities of the alimentary tract, including the pharynx, esophagus, stomach, duodenum, jejunum, ileum, and colon. Additionally falling under the auspices of gastrointestinal radiology is imaging of the accessory organs of the gastrointestinal system, including the liver, biliary system, spleen, and pancreas.

Imaging Modalities

Imaging modalities that are used in gastrointestinal radiology include conventional radiography, fluoroscopy, computed tomography (CT), ultrasonography, magnetic resonance imaging (MRI), and nuclear medicine. **Fluoroscopy** has remained the cornerstone of radiologic imaging of the hollow viscera of the gastrointestinal system (Fig. 1–1) since the 1920s, enduring the emergence of multiple modern imaging modalities. Fluoroscopy permits dynamic evaluation of the alimentary tract.

Because of the dynamic nature of the examinations, radiologist expertise, technologist proficiency, and patient cooperation all are important factors in obtaining optimal diagnostic images. The fluoroscope tabletop can be moved from a completely vertical position (90 degrees), through the horizontal (0 degrees), to a steep head-down position (≤ -45 degrees). Additionally the patient can be placed supine, prone, lateral, or in any degree of obliquity on the fluoroscope tabletop (Table 1–1). Right lateral decubitus and left lateral decubitus positions indicate that the x-ray beam is directed horizontally, with the patient in the right lateral and left lateral positions, respectively.

Fluoroscopic contrast agents are employed to allow visualization of structures that are by themselves essentially radiographically unapparent. The most commonly used contrast agent is **barium sulfate**, an alkaline earth metallic element that is suspended in liquid and used to outline the hollow viscera of the alimentary tract. The density of the barium suspension is quantified using **percent weight volume (% w/v)**, which simply refers to the weight of $BaSO_4$ powder (in grams) added to sufficient volume of water to produce 100 mL.

Single-contrast technique refers to the us-

Table 1–1.
Patient Positions Commonly Referred to in Gastrointestinal Radiology

Name	Abbreviation	Description
Anteroposterior	AP	Supine
Right posterior oblique	RPO	Supine and rotated to the right
Right lateral	RL	Right side down
Right anterior oblique	RAO	Prone and rotated to the right
Posteroanterior	PA	Prone
Left anterior oblique	LAO	Prone and rotated to the left
Left lateral	LL	Left side down
Left posterior oblique	LPO	Supine and rotated to the left

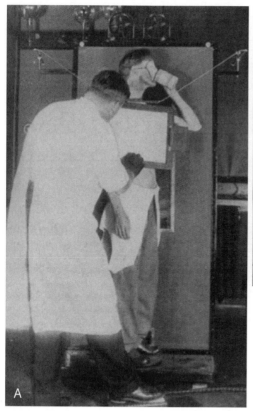

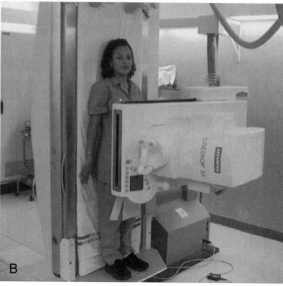

Figure 1–1. Fluoroscopy: then and now. A, Dr. Russel D. Carman (1875–1926), one of the fathers of gastrointestinal fluoroscopy, performing an esophagram in 1917. **B,** A modern fluoroscopy suite. (**A,** From Carman RD, Miller A: The Roentgen Diagnosis of Diseases of the Alimentary Canal. Philadelphia, WB Saunders, 1917.)

age of a dilute barium suspension or water-soluble contrast agent to completely fill a hollow viscus, whereas **double-contrast** technique involves coating the mucosal surface with a dense barium suspension while the organ is distended with gas. **Biphasic** technique refers to a combination of single-contrast and double-contrast techniques that are performed sequentially to achieve the benefits of each type of examination.

Water-soluble contrast agents are iodinated solutions that alternatively can be used for single-contrast technique when there is a suspicion of visceral perforation. In contrast to barium, water-soluble agents are absorbed readily by the body after leakage.

In general, double-contrast examinations are more difficult to perform because they require meticulous technique to coat the entire mucosal surface adequately and distend the organ sufficiently with gas, while avoiding pooling of dense barium, which could obscure areas of pathology. Gaseous distention can be accomplished by insufflation of air or ingestion of effervescent granules. Consequently, these examinations require significantly more patient cooperation

and mobility than single-contrast examinations. Double-contrast examinations often allow greater visualization of subtle mucosal abnormalities that usually are not apparent using single-contrast technique. It often is preferable, however, to perform a more reliable single-contrast examination than a suboptimal double-contrast examination in a patient who is unable to cooperate adequately for the procedure.

Computed tomography is one of the first-line modalities for evaluation of the solid viscera of the gastrointestinal system. As the patient passes through the CT gantry, axial images are constructed as x-rays are passed through the patient to small detectors on the side opposite the x-ray tube. Modern multislice volumetric spiral CT scanners can image the entire abdomen and pelvis during a single breath hold. CT imaging techniques often employ contrast agents to enhance radiographic visualization. Contrast agents include esophageal barium paste, dilute barium suspensions or water-soluble iodinated agents for stomach or bowel opacification, and intravascular water-soluble contrast agents. The bolus of intravascular contrast agent often is administered rapidly by a power injector to ensure optimal tissue enhancement.

Ultrasonography is perhaps the least invasive imaging modality in radiology. Ultrasound beams are produced and received by hand-held transducers that are directed in real time by a sonographer. Because of the limitations of ultrasound to image gas-filled hollow viscera, it has limited applications in gastrointestinal radiology and is used to noninvasively image the solid organs, blood vessels, and biliary system. Ultrasound is often the preferred imaging modality for evaluation of the gallbladder and several pediatric conditions.

Magnetic resonance imaging is a complex imaging modality based on the magnetic characteristics of various tissues, which also is used for evaluation of the solid viscera, blood vessels, and biliary system. Because of its relatively high cost and the ready availability of CT and ultrasound, MRI often serves as an adjunctive imaging modality for gastrointestinal radiology. The primary applications of MRI for the gastrointestinal system include evaluation of liver lesions and magnetic resonance cholangiopancreatography. MRI is useful for patients that cannot undergo contrast-enhanced CT because of renal dysfunction.

Nuclear medicine imaging (scintigraphy) can be used for several specific applications in gastrointestinal radiology. Radionuclides, such as technetium 99m, are complexed to substances such as sulfur colloid, pertechnetate, red blood cells, and iminodiacetic acid analogs, which are administered to the patient. Colloidal liver-spleen imaging is used for evaluation of specific hepatic space-occupying lesions (e.g., hemangioma, hepatic adenoma, and focal nodular hyperplasia) and for localization of splenic tissue. Labeled red blood cell scans are employed for localization of gastrointestinal hemorrhage. Hepatobiliary imaging is used for detecting acute cholecystitis, evaluating biliary patency, and differentiating biliary atresia from neonatal hepatitis. Meckel diverticula can be localized with radiopharmaceuticals. Detection and quantification of gastroesophageal reflux and gastric emptying rates can be performed with nuclear medicine imaging.

Suggested Readings

Gore RM, Levine MS, Laufer I: Textbook of Gastrointestinal Radiology, 2nd ed. Philadelphia, WB Saunders, 2000.

Houston JD, Davis M: Fundamentals of Fluoroscopy. Philadelphia, WB Saunders, 2001.

Mettler FA, Guiberteau MJ: Essentials of Nuclear Medicine Imaging, 4th ed. Philadelphia, WB Saunders, 1998.

Webb WR, Brant WE, Helms CA: Fundamentals of Body CT, 2nd ed. Philadelphia, WB Saunders, 1998.

Williamson SL: Essentials of Pediatric Radiology. Philadelphia, WB Saunders, 2001.

TWO

Pharynx

JEFFREY D. HOUSTON, M.D., AND MICHAEL DAVIS, M.D.

Normal Anatomy

The **pharynx** extends from the oral cavity to the cervical esophagus and is divided into the nasopharynx, oropharynx, and hypopharynx (Fig. 2–1). The **nasopharynx** is the portion of the pharynx posterior to the soft palate that extends from the base of the skull to the tip of the uvula. It functions as a segment of the respiratory tract when the mouth is closed. The nasopharynx is isolated from the alimentary tract during deglutition (swallowing) by elevation of the soft palate. The pharyngeal tonsils (adenoids) and the openings of the eustachian tubes reside in the nasopharynx.

The complex anatomy of the orohypopharynx is shown best using double-contrast technique to coat the pharyngeal contents with dense barium (Fig. 2–2). The **oropharynx** is contained by the space between the tip of the uvula and the hyoid bone. The anterior oropharynx is formed by the base of the tongue and a portion of the epiglottis. The **valleculae** are paired depressions that are located between the base of the tongue and the epiglottis. The middle and inferior pharyngeal constrictor muscles form the lateral and posterior oropharyngeal walls. The oropharynx also contains the palatine tonsils.

The **hypopharynx** (laryngopharynx) is the portion of the pharynx posterior to the larynx that extends through the level of the hyoid bone to the junction of the cervical esophagus. The hypopharynx communicates anteriorly with the larynx through the **laryngeal aditus**. The **aryepiglottic folds** separate the laryngeal aditus from the **piriform recesses**, which are small depressions posterolateral to the larynx. The inferior pharyngeal constrictor muscles form the lateral and posterior walls of the hypopharynx. The **cricopharyngeus muscle** resides at the

level of the C5–6 disk space and is the primary component of the upper esophageal sphincter.

The cartilaginous **epiglottis** tilts posteriorly during deglutition and prevents access to the laryngeal aditus and the trachea. The **larynx** extends between the pharynx and the trachea and is composed of a skeleton of nine cartilages, multiple ligaments, and the true and false vocal cords. The **glottis** consists of the true vocal cords and the aperture between them.

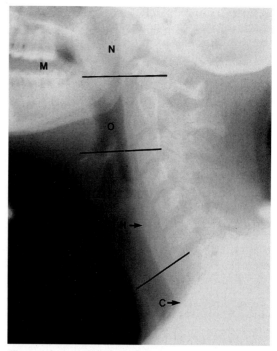

Figure 2–1. Anatomic divisions of the pharynx. Conventional lateral soft tissue neck radiograph shows the anatomic divisions of the pharynx: oral cavity/mouth (M), nasopharynx (N), oropharynx (O), hypopharynx (H), and cervical esophagus (C). (From Houston JD, Davis M: Fundamentals of Fluoroscopy. Philadelphia, WB Saunders, 2001.)

4

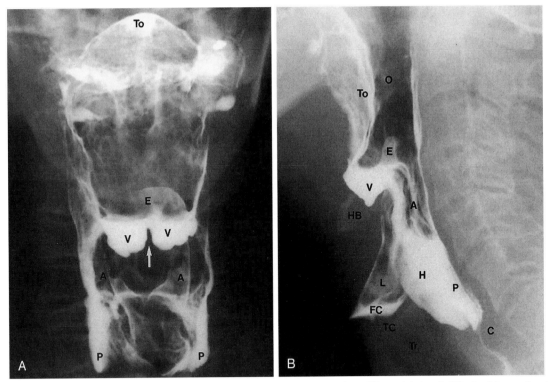

Figure 2–2. Anatomy of the pharynx. Abnormal anteroposterior **(A)** and lateral **(B)** double-contrast pharyngograms allow visualization of pharyngeal anatomy: oropharynx (O), base of tongue (To), epiglottis (E), valleculae (V), piriform recesses (P), aryepiglottic folds (A), hyoid bone (HB), hypopharynx (H), larynx (L), false cords (FC), true cords (TC), trachea (Tr), and cricopharyngeus muscle (C). (From Houston JD, Davis M: Fundamentals of Fluoroscopy. Philadelphia, WB Saunders, 2001.)

Swallowing is a complex mechanism that is controlled by multiple muscles and nerves (Fig. 2–3). The oral phase begins with sizing and mastication, after which the bolus is transferred by a muscular wave within the tongue into the back of the mouth. The bolus is propelled into the oropharynx by thrusting of the tongue, while nasopharyngeal reflux is prevented by a seal that is created by apposition of the soft palate to a more muscular segment of the posterior pharyngeal wall known as the **Passavant cushion** or **pad**. Aided by gravity, sequential muscular contractions propel the bolus through the orohypopharynx. The larynx elevates in conjunction with tilting of the epiglottis to protect the airway. The upper esophageal sphincter relaxes and allows passage of the bolus into the cervical esophagus. Swallowing is under voluntary control by striated muscle until the bolus reaches the level of the aortic arch, where involuntary smooth muscle engages the bolus. The esophageal primary contraction wave then propels it to the lower esophageal sphincter, which opens and allows the bolus to enter the stomach.

Imaging Modalities

Indications for radiologic examination of the pharynx include **dysphagia** (difficulty swallowing); **odynophagia** (painful swallowing); **globus** (sensation of a lump in the throat); suspected aspiration, foreign body, epiglottitis, or abscess; and after blunt or penetrating trauma. Radiologic examination of the pharynx can be performed using conventional radiographs, single-contrast or double-contrast pharyngography, and computed tomography (CT). Conventional radiographs generally are used for evaluating for epiglottitis, pharyngeal edema, retropharyngeal abscesses, and radiopaque foreign bodies.

Contrasted videofluoroscopic examinations are best suited for evaluating functional swallowing abnormalities. When employing single-contrast technique, video

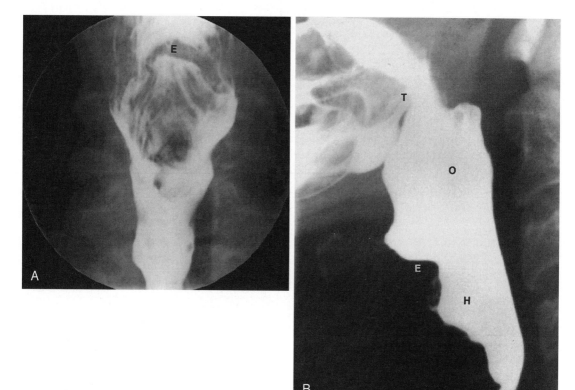

Figure 2–3. Pharyngogram during deglutition. Normal anteroposterior **(A)** and lateral **(B)** single-contrast pharyngograms during deglutition show distention of the pharynx with barium, posterior tilting of the epiglottis, and the expected obliteration of many anatomic landmarks. Visualized structures include: base of tongue (T), oropharynx (O), epiglottis (E), and hypopharynx (H). (From Houston JD, Davis M: Fundamentals of Fluoroscopy. Philadelphia, WB Saunders, 2001.)

recording is essential to capture the dynamics of deglutition. The video recorder should have freeze-frame capability so that abnormalities can be studied in detail. If hard copy images are needed, rapid spot filming with a high-speed camera or a digital fluoroscopy unit may be performed. If patients are unable to stand or sit on the footboard of the fluoroscopy table, a C-arm fluoroscope can be used while the patient is sitting in a wheelchair or lying on a stretcher with the head elevated. Examinations should be performed in the anteroposterior and lateral projections. Swallowing studies often are performed in conjunction with speech pathologists, who can observe the dynamics of swallowing using food substances of varying textures and consistencies, while employing different maneuvers to improve swallowing.

Functional Abnormalities

Functional abnormalities of the pharynx that can be seen on fluoroscopic swallowing examinations include abnormal oral transit, inadequate propulsion of the bolus (retention), **nasopharyngeal reflux** (Fig. 2–4), pooling in the valleculae or piriform sinuses (Fig. 2–5), **laryngeal penetration** (to the level of the false cords), and frank **tracheal aspiration** (to the level of the true cords or below). Barium should be used as the contrast agent in patients who may aspirate because ionic water-soluble contrast material can result in pulmonary edema. Severe aspiration can result in barium outlining the tracheobronchial tree (Fig. 2–6). Abnormalities of the cricopharyngeus muscle, such as **cricopharyngeal achalasia** (failure of relaxation) or **cricopharyngeal hypertrophy** (Fig. 2–7), also can result in dysphagia.

Structural Abnormalities

Benign pharyngeal **strictures** may result from surgery, trauma, iatrogenic injury (e.g.,

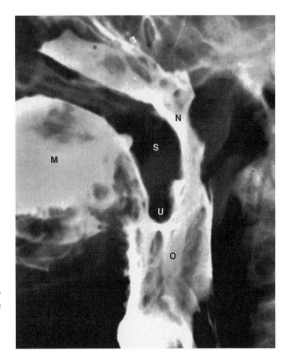

Figure 2–4. Nasopharyngeal reflux. Lateral single-contrast pharyngogram demonstrates filling of the mouth (M) and oropharynx (O) with barium as well as massive reflux into the nasopharynx (N). Barium outlines the soft palate (S) and uvula (U).

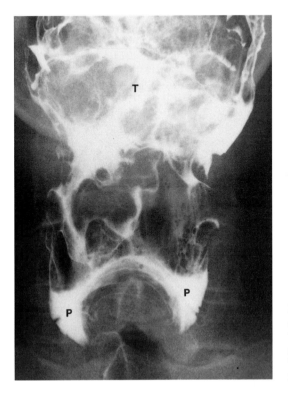

Figure 2–5. Pharyngeal paresis. Single-contrast anteroposterior pharyngogram reveals pooling in the piriform sinuses (P) in a patient with pharyngeal paresis. Residual barium on the base of the tongue (T) allows visualization of numerous round filling defects, representing lingual papillae.

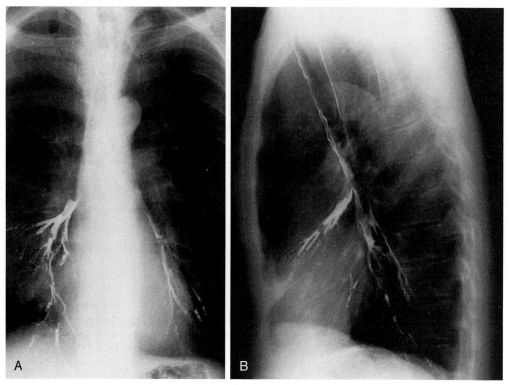

Figure 2–6. Severe aspiration. Barium outlines the dependent portions of the tracheobronchial tree on frontal **(A)** and lateral **(B)** chest radiographs.

endoscopy), caustic chemical ingestion, and irradiation (Fig. 2–8). Pharyngeal **webs** are thin mucosal folds that either partly or completely encircle the pharynx. They usually are insignificant and are seen occasionally in patients without symptoms. They usually are found on the anterior wall of the hypopharynx near the junction of the cervical esophagus (Fig. 2–9). Webs generally appear as 1- to 2-mm thin linear, horizontally oriented persistent filling defects. Webs can be confused with prominent submucosal ve-

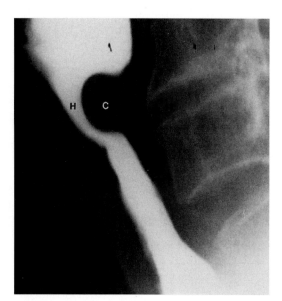

Figure 2–7. Cricopharyngeal hypertrophy. Lateral single-contrast pharyngogram displays prominence of the cricopharyngeus muscle (C), which significantly narrows the adjacent hypopharynx (H) anteriorly.

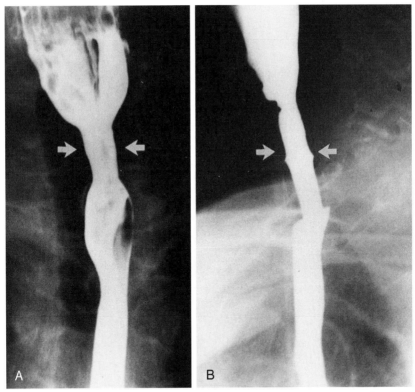

Figure 2–8. Benign stricture. Anteroposterior **(A)** and lateral **(B)** single-contrast pharyngograms reveal a long segment of narrowing of the pharynx from a benign stricture *(arrows)*.

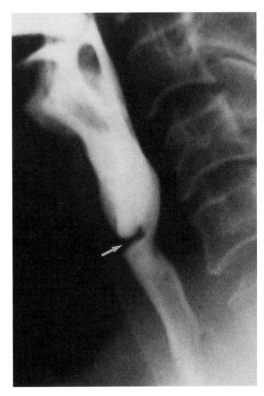

Figure 2–9. Pharyngeal web. A thin shelf-like ridge of tissue *(arrow)* emanates from the anterior pharyngeal wall and is outlined by barium on this lateral single-contrast pharyngogram.

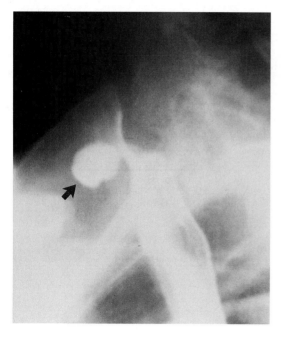

Figure 2–10. Pharyngeal diverticulum. Filling of an anterior outpouching of the pharynx *(arrow)* with barium is documented by a single-contrast pharyngogram.

nous plexuses, which generally are triangular and dynamic.

Diverticula of the pharynx are occasionally encountered outpouchings of the wall that generally are acquired (Fig. 2–10). True diverticula contain all the normal layers of the wall, whereas false diverticula generally consist of only mucosa, which herniates through a muscular defect.

The **Zenker (pharyngoesophageal) diverticulum** represents herniation of mucosa through the posterolateral aspect of the hypopharynx, just above the cricopharyngeus muscle. Herniation occurs through an anatomic zone of sparse musculature known as the **Killian dehiscence**. The pharyngeal mucosa herniates through this zone of weak musculature owing to a high-pressure gradi-

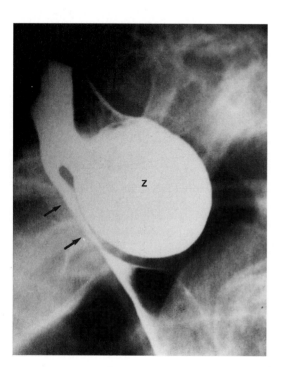

Figure 2–11. Zenker diverticulum. Lateral single-contrast pharyngogram illustrates filling of a large Zenker diverticulum (Z), which exerts mass effect on the more anterior cervical esophagus *(arrows)*.

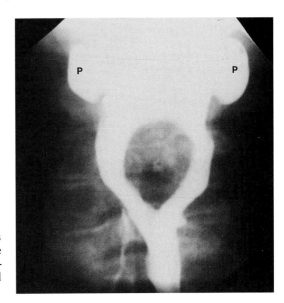

Figure 2–12. Lateral pharyngeal pouches. Pouches (P) arising from the lateral pharyngeal walls are seen transiently on this anteroposterior single-contrast pharyngogram while the pharynx is distended with barium.

ent caused by a hyperactive cricopharyngeal sphincter. Over time, the mucosal herniation becomes a diverticulum. If a diverticulum becomes large enough, it can compress the pharynx and esophagus and cause dysphagia (Fig. 2–11).

A rare site of hypopharyngeal diverticulum formation is laterally, in the **Killian-Jamison space**, which is located between the cricopharyngeus muscle and the proximal longitudinal fibers of the esophagus. This space represents the site of entry of the recurrent laryngeal nerve and associated blood vessels.

Lateral pharyngeal pouches (pharyngoceles) are acquired bulges in the lateral walls of the hypopharynx at an area of anatomic weakness in the anterolateral aspect of the piriform sinuses (Fig. 2–12). They are seen commonly, are often bilaterally symmetric, and are usually of no clinical significance. Pharyngoceles are reported to be associated with horn players and glass blowers because of the increased intraluminal pressure stemming from these activities. Rare **lateral pharyngeal diverticula** have a similar appearance to the lateral pharyngeal pouches but can be differentiated by their persistent bulges, whereas the bulges from pharyngoceles are seen only transiently during pharyngeal distention.

The **laryngocele** is a rarely encountered dilation of the appendix of the laryngeal ventricle that can herniate through the thyrohyoid ligament into the soft tissues of the neck. Because of their location, laryngoceles nor-

mally are not filled with barium on pharyngograms.

Pharyngitis

Retropharyngeal abscesses can result from penetrating trauma, dental disease, and pharyngitis. Radiographic findings include widening of the retropharyngeal space and gas in the parapharyngeal soft tissues (Fig. 2–13). Posterior pharyngeal wall thickening can be secondary to edema, hematoma, or other soft tissue masses (Fig. 2–14).

Epiglottitis results from inflammation of the epiglottis, most commonly secondary to *Haemophilus influenzae* (Fig. 2–15). It generally occurs in children, but occasionally can occur in adults. Epiglottitis is a medical emergency that should be diagnosed with a conventional radiograph of the neck using soft tissue technique or indirect laryngoscopy because manipulation of the epiglottis can result in abrupt loss of control of the airway.

Extrinsic deformity of the pharynx can result from any space-occupying lesion of the neck. Lymphadenopathy, thyroid enlargement, cysts, neoplasms, and anterior cervical spine osteophytes can deform the pharynx extrinsically (Fig. 2–16).

Benign Neoplasms

Benign tumors of the pharynx are uncommon. Neoplasms originating from the sur-

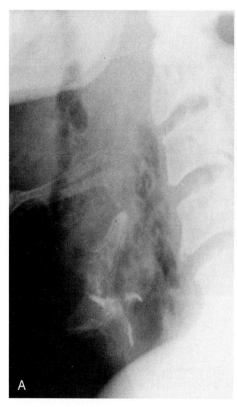

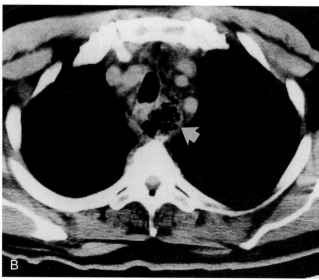

Figure 2–13. Retropharyngeal abscess. A, Lateral neck radiograph reveals bubbly lucencies from gas throughout the soft tissues surrounding the pharynx in a patient with a retropharyngeal abscess. **B,** Gas is observed to dissect inferiorly into the mediastinum *(arrow)* on an axial CT image. Soft tissue air can be seen after traumatic perforation of the pharynx or can be seen dissecting superiorly from a tracheal or esophageal injury.

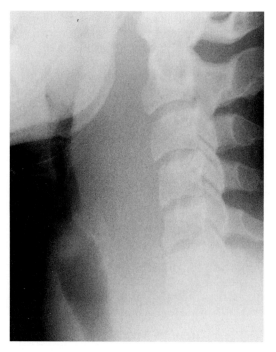

Figure 2–14. Retropharyngeal edema. Lateral neck radiograph demonstrates severe thickening of the prevertebral soft tissues from edema.

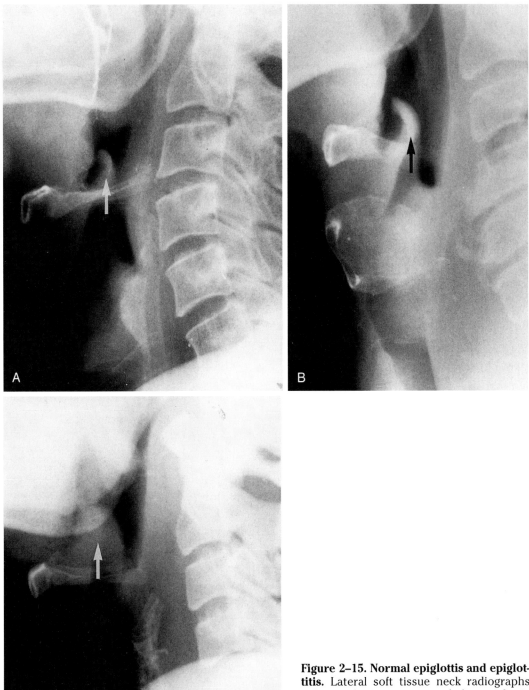

Figure 2–15. Normal epiglottis and epiglottitis. Lateral soft tissue neck radiographs indicate the appearance of the epiglottis *(arrows)* in a normal patient **(A)**, contrasted to the thickened edematous appearances in mild **(B)** and severe epiglottitis **(C)**.

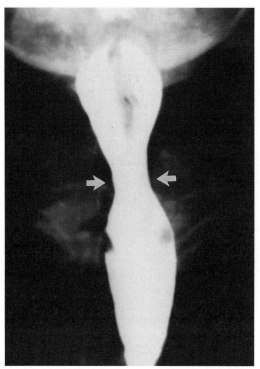

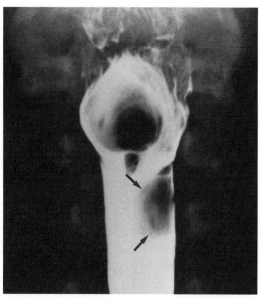

Figure 2–17. Epithelial cyst. Anteroposterior single-contrast pharyngogram reveals a unilateral rounded filling defect of the left pharynx *(arrows)*, representing an epithelial cyst.

Figure 2–16. Extrinsic pharyngeal narrowing. Anteroposterior single-contrast pharyngogram displays extrinsic mass effect on the pharynx *(arrows)* from thyromegaly.

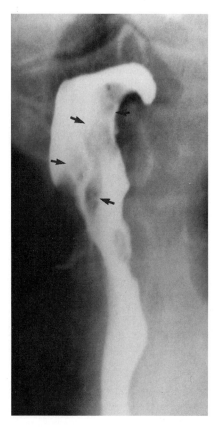

Figure 2–18. Squamous cell carcinoma. Lateral single-contrast pharyngogram reveals irregular filling defects *(arrows)* and luminal narrowing of the distal pharynx and proximal esophagus resulting from a very large squamous cell carcinoma.

face and glandular epithelium include papillomas and cysts (Fig. 2–17). Neoplasms of mesenchymal origin include fibromas, hemangiomas, and angiofibromas. Radiographic features of pharyngeal neoplasms include round filling defects and luminal deviation.

Malignant Neoplasms

Squamous cell carcinoma accounts for most malignant tumors of the pharynx and is associated with alcohol and tobacco abuse. Patients with Plummer-Vinson syndrome are at increased risk of developing pharyngeal carcinoma. Squamous cell carcinomas may arise from the palatine tonsil, base of the tongue, epiglottis, piriform sinuses, and valleculae. Synchronous esophageal carcinomas have been reported in a few patients with squamous cell carcinoma of the pharynx.

Lymphoma and multiple rare tumors, such as adenocarcinoma, melanoma, and sarcoma, constitute the remainder of malignant pharyngeal neoplasms. Radiographic features of malignant pharyngeal neoplasms include irregular filling defects, strictures, luminal deviation, soft tissue thickening, and ulcerations (Fig. 2–18).

Suggested Readings

Gore RM, Levine MS, Laufer I: Textbook of Gastrointestinal Radiology, 2nd ed. Philadelphia, WB Saunders, 2000.

Houston JD, Davis M: Fundamentals of Fluoroscopy. Philadelphia, WB Saunders, 2001.

Levine MS: Radiology of the Esophagus. Philadelphia, WB Saunders, 1989.

THREE

Esophagus

MICHAEL DAVIS, M.D., AND JEFFREY D. HOUSTON, M.D.

Normal Anatomy

The esophagus consists of cervical and thoracic segments as well as a small abdominal component. The short **cervical esophagus** begins at the pharyngoesophageal junction near C5–6 and extends to the thoracic inlet. The **thoracic esophagus** comprises most of the esophagus and is divided arbitrarily into supra-aortic, bronchial, retrocardiac, and epiphrenic segments. Normal extrinsic impressions on the esophagus include the aortic arch and the left main stem bronchus (Fig. 3–1).

The cervical and thoracic portions of the esophagus constitute the **tubular esophagus**. The **esophageal vestibule** represents an area of saccular dilation of the terminal thoracic esophagus. The tubulovestibular junction is referred to as the *A-level*. The vestibule is bounded distally by the gastroesophageal junction, or the *B-level*. The **esophageal hiatus** is the opening in the left hemidiaphragm through which the esophagus passes into the abdomen. The **lower esophageal sphincter** (LES) encompasses the abdominal segment of the esophagus and functions to prevent reflux of gastric contents into the esophagus.

The esophageal lumen normally is lined by stratified squamous epithelium. The **Z-line** represents the zigzagging abrupt transition zone to the simple columnar epithelium of the stomach (Fig. 3–2).

Two types of peristaltic waves normally result in the movement of a bolus through the esophagus. The **primary contraction wave** is initiated by swallowing, when the cervical esophagus is distended by a bolus. The **secondary contraction wave** results from a bolus in the thoracic esophagus, with the purpose of clearing any residual luminal contents remaining after the primary wave. Normal contraction waves have an inverted V-shaped pattern of progressive obliteration of the esophageal lumen and are followed by a wave of relaxation.

Imaging Modalities

Common indications for contrast examination of the esophagus include dysphagia, odynophagia, pyrosis (heartburn), substernal chest pain, midepigastric pain, symptoms indicative of esophageal obstruction, or a sensation of food lodging in the esophagus. Esophagography can be performed with single-contrast or double-contrast technique.

Single-contrast esophagography is used to evaluate esophageal patency, extrinsic abnormalities (e.g., vascular anomalies, mediastinal adenopathy, and neoplasms), cardiac chamber enlargement, stricture, and hiatal hernia. Mucosal detail is evaluated poorly with this technique. The examination generally is performed with the patient in the right anterior oblique position to offset the esophagus from the spine, with the head of the tabletop declined to −15 degrees to promote maximal distention of the esophagus. Medium-density barium (50% to 60% weight volume [w/v]) is sipped continually with a straw while images of the entire esophagus are obtained (Fig. 3–3A). Water-soluble contrast material should be used if there is a suspicion of esophageal perforation because, in contrast to barium, it is absorbed by the soft tissues. Water-soluble contrast material should be avoided if there is a suspicion of aspiration or a tracheoesophageal fistula because it can result in pulmonary edema.

Double-contrast esophagography shows fine mucosal detail from subtle abnormalities, such as early inflammatory changes of reflux disease or infectious esophagitis. Early tumor formation can be detected in

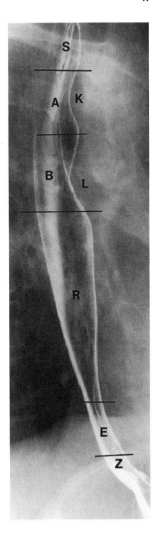

Figure 3–1. Normal anatomy of the esophagus. Normal impressions on the aorta are the aortic knob (K) and left main stem bronchus (L). Anatomic segments of the aorta are: supra-aortic segment (S) from the thoracic inlet to the aortic arch, aortic arch segment (A) through the aortic arch to the carina, bronchial segment (B) from the carina through the left main stem bronchus, retrocardiac segment (R) from the left main stem bronchus to the left lateral deviation, epiphrenic segment (E) from the left lateral deviation to esophageal hiatus, and sphincter zone (Z) from the esophageal hiatus to the gastroesophageal junction. (From Houston JD, Davis M: Fundamentals of Fluoroscopy. Philadelphia, WB Saunders, 2001.)

this manner. This examination generally is performed with the patient standing on the footboard of the fluoroscopy table in the left posterior oblique position to offset the esophagus from the spine. Effervescent granules are swallowed to distend the esophagus with gas, followed by dense barium (200% to 250% w/v) to coat the mucosa while images of the entire esophagus are obtained (Fig. 3–3B).

Computed tomography (CT) has limited utility in the diagnosis of esophageal disorders because of nondistention of the lumen, but is useful for evaluation for extension of esophageal disease and its relationship to adjacent structures (Fig. 3–4). If an esophageal mass is identified, further evaluation can be performed with contrast-enhanced CT and esophageal paste (3% w/v) to evaluate for local invasion, lymphadenopathy, and other metastatic disease.

Gastroesophageal scintigraphy can be used to detect and quantify gastroesophageal reflux. The patient ingests a mixture of technetium 99m–labeled sulfur colloid and hydrochloric acid diluted in orange juice, after which sequential images are obtained while abdominal pressure is increased incrementally using an abdominal binder. This examination is more sensitive for detecting reflux than fluoroscopy, but lacks the ability to show the detrimental effects of gastroesophageal reflux disease on the esophagus. Gastroesophageal reflux often is not elucidated fluoroscopically in patients with proven reflux esophagitis.

Functional Abnormalities

Motility disorders of the esophagus include proximal escape, tertiary contraction

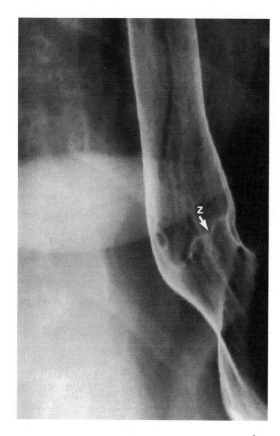

Figure 3–2. Z-line. The zigzagging squamosal-columnar mucosal junction (Z) is seen in this double-contrast esophagram. (From Houston JD, Davis M: Fundamentals of Fluoroscopy. Philadelphia, WB Saunders, 2001.)

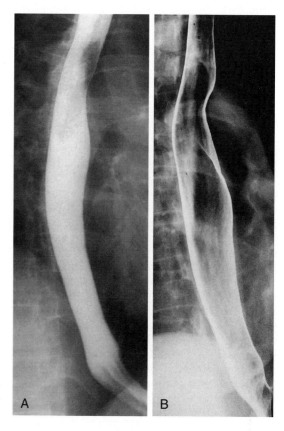

Figure 3–3. Normal esophagography. Normal single-contrast **(A)** and double-contrast **(B)** esophagrams.

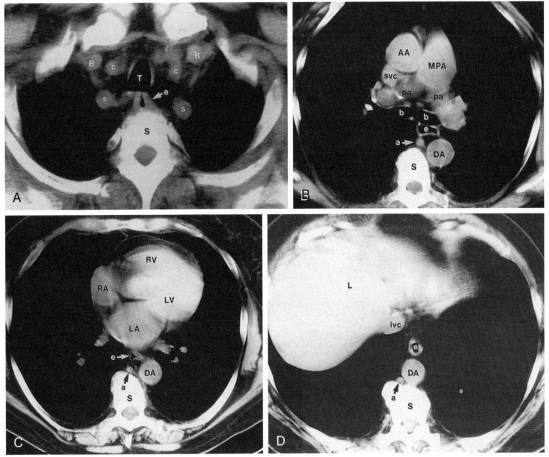

Figure 3–4. Normal CT of the esophagus. Sequential noncontrasted axial CT images **(A–D)** show the relationship of the esophagus (e) to adjacent structures in the thorax and abdomen: trachea (T), spine (S), carotid arteries (c), brachiocephalic veins (B), subclavian arteries (s), ascending aorta (AA), descending aorta (DA), main pulmonary artery (MPA), pulmonary arteries (pa), bronchi (b), superior vena cava (svc), azygos vein (a), right atrium (RA), right ventricle (RV), left ventricle (LV), left atrium (LA), liver (L), and inferior vena cava (ivc).

waves, presbyesophagus, achalasia, and progressive systemic sclerosis. Esophageal motility disorders are controversial with regard to the suspected cause and recommended treatment.

A common motility disorder in the proximal esophagus is referred to as **proximal escape,** "elevator esophagus," or "to-and-fro" peristalsis. At fluoroscopy, the primary wave pushing the barium bolus caudally often "breaks" at the junction of the proximal and middle thirds with regression of the barium bolus proximally. Patients with this disorder often complain of a feeling of tightness in the throat at the level of the suprasternal

notch. The cause of this common motility disorder is unknown.

Tertiary (nonpropulsive) contraction waves result from contraction of the muscularis propria and are neither propagated throughout the esophagus nor followed by a receptive wave of relaxation. Radiographically, these waves appear as indentations at the margins of the esophagus that occur over local or large segments of the esophagus (Fig. 3–5). Tertiary contractions can be represented as deep indentations of the esophagus. The frequency of tertiary waves increases with aging.

Transient transversely oriented mucosal

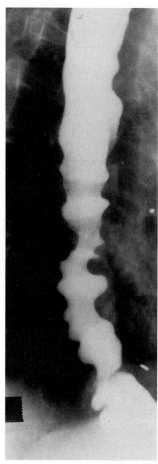

Figure 3–5. Esophageal spasm. Single-contrast esophagram reveals deep tertiary contractions in the distal third of the esophagus.

tions that follow at least 30% of swallows and are interspersed with normal peristaltic waves. Radiographically, this condition appears as a **corkscrew esophagus** (Fig. 3–8). Patients suffer from chest pain or dysphagia, particularly after ingesting cold or hot liquids.

Achalasia of the esophagus is a relatively common insidious disorder resulting from incomplete relaxation of the LES because of neuronal degeneration, which causes hypoperistalsis or aperistalsis of the body of the esophagus. It is manifested radiographically by dilation of the esophagus (often containing an air-fluid level), which sometimes originally is detected incidentally on chest radiographs (Fig. 3–9). With time, the esophagus becomes markedly dilated. Esophagography reveals a normal peristaltic wave ad-

folds can be observed occasionally in the esophagus, representing contraction of the longitudinally oriented muscularis mucosa. Because transverse folds are seen normally in cats, this appearance is termed **feline esophagus** (Fig. 3–6). These folds can be a normal variant, may occur in progressive systemic sclerosis (scleroderma), or can be a response to gastroesophageal reflux.

Presbyesophagus is an asymptomatic disorder of motor function occurring in older individuals. Hallmarks of presbyesophagus include failure of a primary peristaltic wave to pass completely through the esophagus to the stomach, tertiary contractions in response to swallowing, aperistalsis, and either an absence of contraction of the LES or failure of relaxation with swallowing (Fig. 3–7).

Diffuse esophageal spasm is characterized by severe repetitive tertiary contrac-

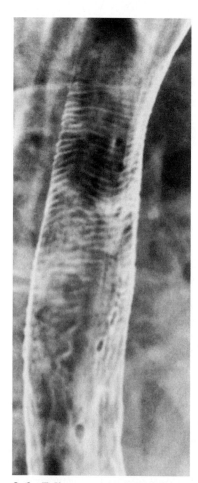

Figure 3–6. Feline esophagus. Double-contrast esophagram demonstrates fine, wavy, horizontal lines in the esophagus, consistent with contraction of the muscularis mucosa.

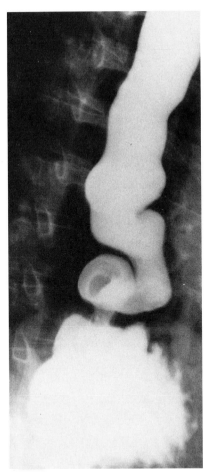

submucosally, causing stricture of this area with proximal dilation of the body at the esophagus. The degree of esophageal dilation is usually less than that seen in true achalasia. **Chagas disease** (American trypanosomiasis) is caused by the protozoan parasite *Trypanosoma cruzi*, which infects and destroys the myenteric plexuses of the esophagus and colon and causes myocarditis and cardiac aneurysms. Chagas disease is seen mostly in South America, Central America, and southern Mexico.

Progressive systemic sclerosis (scleroderma) is a systemic disorder of abnormally increased fibrosis. Progressive muscular atrophy with resulting collagen deposition can involve the entire gastrointestinal tract, but particularly the distal two thirds of the esophagus. Esophageal involvement is mani-

Figure 3–7. Presbyesophagus. Single-contrast esophagram displays the *curling phenomenon* often seen in elderly patients with presbyesophagus.

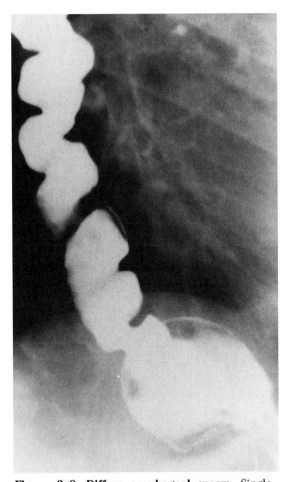

Figure 3–8. Diffuse esophageal spasm. Single-contrast esophagram illustrates severe tertiary contractions that give the esophagus a *corkscrew* appearance.

vancing to the thoracic inlet but not beyond. The barium falls by gravity to the LES, which has a beaklike appearance that relaxes only momentarily (Fig. 3–10). There is an increased incidence of squamous cell carcinoma of the esophagus in patients with achalasia.

Primary achalasia is diagnosed when no underlying disease is present. The cause remains controversial, but there is degeneration of the myenteric plexus that disrupts the neuromuscular transmission that signals the LES to open normally.

Secondary achalasia (pseudoachalasia) refers to the functional changes of achalasia that occur in the setting of underlying conditions, such as neoplasms or Chagas disease. Secondary achalasia usually is secondary to gastric cancer that has infiltrated the LES

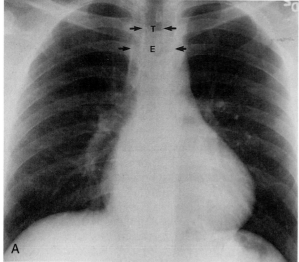

Figure 3–9. Achalasia. Posteroanterior **(A)** and lateral **(B)** chest radiographs in a patient with primary achalasia display two columns of air, representing a normal trachea (T) and an abnormal air-filled dilated esophagus (E).

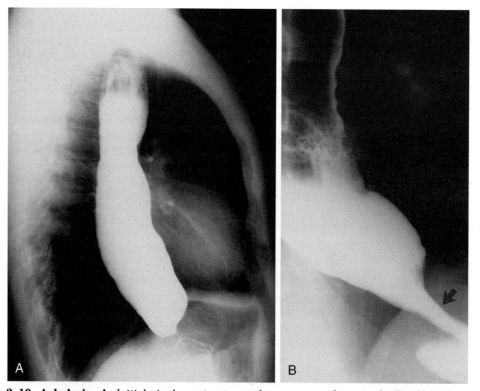

Figure 3–10. Achalasia. A, Initial single-contrast esophagram reveals a markedly dilated esophagus with abrupt narrowing of the distal segment. **B,** Seconds later, the lower esophageal sphincter transiently opens, allowing passage of a small amount of barium and illustrating the beaklike narrowing of the distal esophagus *(arrow).*

fested as absent peristalsis of the smooth muscle and failure of the LES to close properly. With time, distal esophageal strictures and other sequelae of gastroesophageal reflux occur (see Barrett esophagus).

Structural Abnormalities

Esophageal atresia with or without **tracheoesophageal fistula** is the most common congenital abnormality of the esophagus. Many affected infants also have other congenital abnormalities, most commonly of the VACTERL association (*v*ertebral abnormalities, *a*nal atresia, *c*ardiac abnormalities, *tr*acheoesophageal fistula/*e*sophageal atresia, *r*enal agenesis and dysplasia, and *l*imb defects). Coiling of an orogastric tube in the proximal esophagus suggests esophageal atresia. Combined with a gasless abdomen, this finding indicates the absence of a tracheoesophageal fistula (Fig. 3–11).

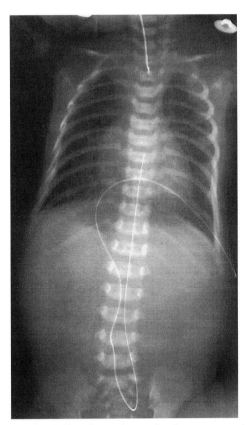

Figure 3–11. Esophageal atresia. Anteroposterior babygram exhibits the inability to place an orogastric tube as well as an entirely gasless abdomen, indicating lack of a tracheoesophageal fistula. (From Williamson SL: Essentials of Pediatric Radiology. Philadelphia, WB Saunders, 2001.)

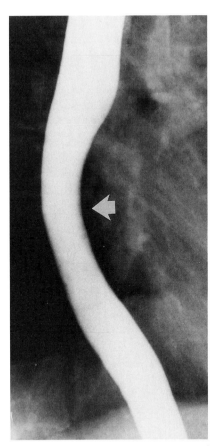

Figure 3–12. Left atrial enlargement. Single-contrast esophagram displays anterior compression of the esophagus *(arrow)* from an enlarged left atrium.

Acquired vascular abnormalities that can cause extrinsic impression on the esophagus include tortuosity and ectasia of the aorta, thoracic aortic aneurysms, and cardiac chamber enlargement (Fig. 3–12). Mediastinal lymphadenopathy, pulmonary malignancy, and mediastinal lymphoma may impinge on the esophagus, often to a remarkable degree.

Congenital abnormalities of the great vessels, known as "rings and slings," produce extrinsic impressions on the esophagus. The most common **vascular rings** are the double aortic arch and the right aortic arch with an aberrant left subclavian artery (Fig. 3–13). The **aberrant left subclavian artery** arises as the last branch of a right aortic arch and usually passes behind the esophagus to ascend on the left. The opposite of this condition is the **aberrant right subclavian artery,** which arises as the last branch of a left aortic arch and usually

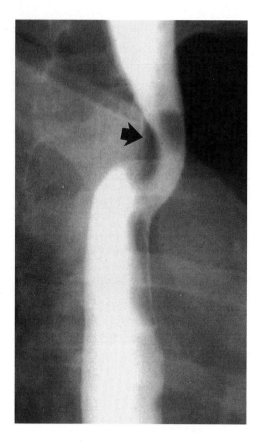

Figure 3–13. Vascular ring. Single-contrast esophagram reveals a posterior impression on the esophagus *(arrow)* from an aberrant right subclavian artery.

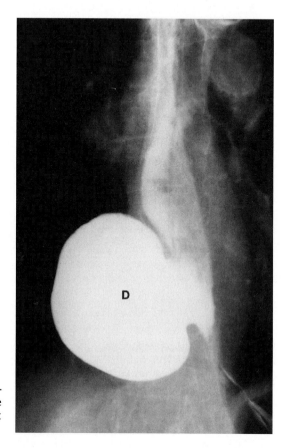

Figure 3–14. Esophageal diverticulum. Single-contrast esophagram illustrates filling of a large epiphrenic diverticulum (D) arising from the right lateral wall of the esophagus.

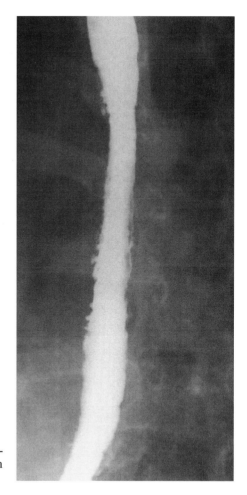

Figure 3–15. Pseudodiverticulosis. Single-contrast esophagram allows filling of intramural pseudodiverticula, which are oriented perpendicular to the esophageal lumen.

passes behind the esophagus to ascend on the right. A **pulmonary sling** occurs when the left pulmonary artery arises from the right pulmonary artery and passes posteriorly and to the left, between the trachea and the esophagus.

Diverticula are common and usually are seen in the midesophagus to lower esophagus. Early literature referred to midesophageal diverticula as *traction* diverticula from mediastinal diseases such as tuberculosis or tumor with or without radiation treatment. Currently, most midesophageal diverticula are of the *pulsion* type. Epiphrenic diverticula may be large (Fig. 3–14) and usually are secondary to a distal esophageal stricture. **Pseudodiverticulosis** of the esophagus is relatively uncommon and represents dilated submucosal glands of the esophagus in the presence of infection (particularly candidiasis) or inflammation (Fig. 3–15).

Hiatal hernias are abnormal herniations of the stomach through the esophageal hiatus of the diaphragm. Hiatal hernias can be divided into two types: sliding (99%) and paraesophageal (1%). In the **sliding hiatal hernia**, the gastroesophageal junction slides superiorly into the chest (Fig. 3–16A). In the rare **paraesophageal hernia**, a portion of the stomach protrudes through the hiatus alongside the esophagus, while the gastroesophageal junction remains normally located below the diaphragm (Fig. 3–16B). Mixed sliding-paraesophageal hernias are extremely rare.

Sliding hiatal hernias can be manifested in many ways with esophagography. Typically, gastric folds are seen rising above the esophageal hiatus. These hernias may be small, may be observed fluoroscopically to slide dynamically above and below the diaphragm, or may be large with a major portion of the stomach being intrathoracic.

Classically, there are several areas of focal narrowing of the distal esophagus, termed **rings**, that are associated with sliding hiatal

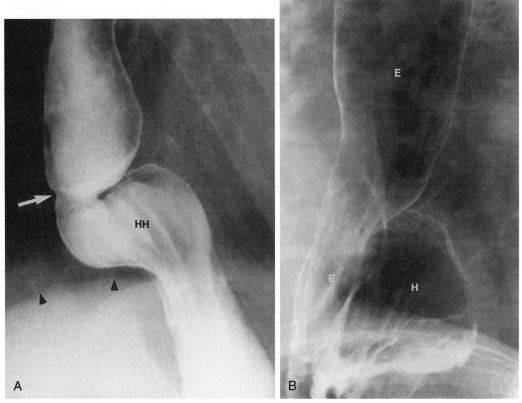

Figure 3–16. Hiatal hernias. A, Single-contrast esophagram reveals gastric folds rising above the diaphragm *(arrowheads)* to the gastroesophageal junction *(arrow)*, representing a sliding hiatal hernia (HH). **B,** Double-contrast esophagram shows a paraesophageal hernia (H), with herniation of the gastric fundus protruding through the esophageal hiatus alongside the esophagus (E).

hernias. The **A-ring** (muscular/contractile ring) represents a broad smooth ring in the region of the tubulovestibular junction that can be observed to change dynamically in caliber (Fig. 3–17A). The **B-ring** (mucosal ring) represents the ridge of tissue at the squamosal-columnar junction. The **Schatzki ring** represents a pathologic B-ring that can result in dysphagia (Fig. 3–17B). It generally is accepted that the B-ring has undergone inflammatory changes from gastroesophageal reflux, causing the ring to become thickened with varying degrees of ensuing narrowing of the esophageal lumen. Almost all rings less than 11 mm (and occasionally 20 mm) in diameter are symptomatic.

Reflux esophagitis is the most common inflammatory disease of the esophagus (Fig. 3–18). Changes of esophagitis begin with limited distensibility, followed by nodularity, thickened folds, erosions, small ulcerations, and stricture. **Barrett esophagus** is an acquired premalignant condition in which pro-

gressive columnar metaplasia replaces the squamous epithelial lining of the distal esophagus with gastric-type epithelium in response to long-standing gastroesophageal reflux. Barrett esophagus forms strictures mostly in the distal esophagus, but short-length, more proximal strictures can also represent Barrett strictures.

Barrett esophagus accounts for many adenocarcinomas in the body of the esophagus and most adenocarcinomas of the gastric cardia, the area that bridges the distal esophagus and proximal stomach. When Barrett esophagus has been established by endoscopic biopsy, surveillance for development of adenocarcinoma is performed periodically with endoscopy and biopsy.

Surgical intervention may be required for treatment of severe gastroesophageal reflux disease. Commonly performed surgeries include the Nissen and Toupet **fundoplications**, Belsey Mark IV repair, and Hill posterior gastropexy. These procedures involve

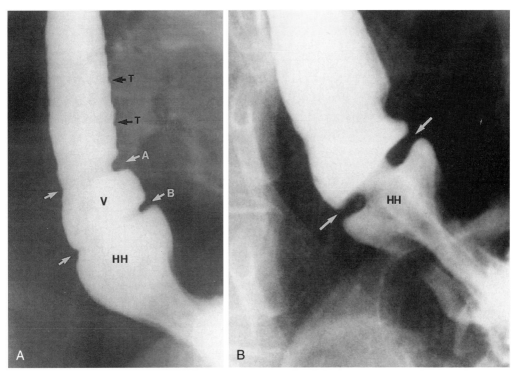

Figure 3–17. Esophageal rings. A, Single-contrast esophagram displays two circumferential filling defects of the distal esophagus. The broader upper ring represents the A-ring (A), and the lower ring represents the B-ring (B). The presence of both rings allows easy visualization of the boundaries of the esophageal vestibule (V) and proves the existence of a sliding hiatal hernia (HH). Note the tertiary contraction wave (T) in the distal esophagus. **B,** Pathologic thickening of the B-ring results in a symptomatic Schatzki ring *(arrows)* in another patient with a sliding hiatal hernia (HH). (**A,** From Houston JD, Davis M: Fundamentals of Fluoroscopy. Philadelphia, WB Saunders, 2001.)

reduction of the hiatal hernia, restoration of the abdominal segment of the esophagus, and wrapping varying degrees of the gastric fundus around the distal esophagus to hinder gastroesophageal reflux (Fig. 3–19).

Infectious Esophagitides

The main infectious diseases of the esophagus are candidiasis, herpes simplex virus, cytomegalovirus, and human immunodeficiency virus (HIV). These conditions often have characteristic radiographic appearances.

Esophageal candidiasis results from the yeast *Candida albicans*. It most commonly presents as "shaggy" mucosa, in which exudate from the yeast forms in a longitudinal linear fashion (Fig. 3–20*A*). Ulcers may occur in candidiasis, but they are difficult to see when there is diffuse disease.

Herpes esophagitis arises from the herpes simplex type I virus and presents radiographically as discrete ulcers, often with a halo of edema, that may be few in number or may be extensive (Fig. 3–20*B*). Herpes ulcers usually are small.

Cytomegalovirus esophagitis often forms large ulcerations that are larger than those caused by herpes, but usually smaller than the giant HIV ulcer (Fig. 3–20*C*). The esophagus may return to normal after treatment of infection, but the potential for stricture formation exists with all esophageal infections.

HIV esophagitis can result in the largest esophageal ulcerations (Fig. 3–20*D*). Because of immunosuppression, patients with acquired immunodeficiency syndrome (AIDS) are at increased risk of developing these infectious esophagitides, particularly cytomegalovirus and *C. albicans*.

Other Esophagitides

Drug-induced esophagitis is common and is represented radiographically as one or more focal ulcerations, usually in the proxi-

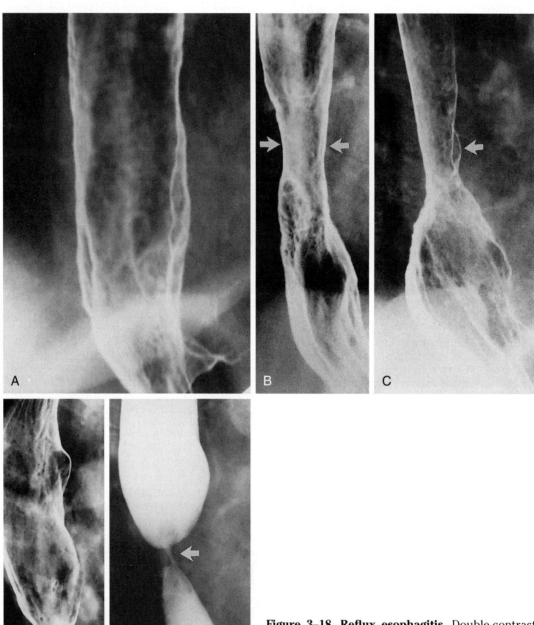

Figure 3–18. Reflux esophagitis. Double-contrast esophagrams show the advancing changes of reflux esophagitis: thickened distal folds with mucosal nodularity **(A)**, slight narrowing of the distal esophagus *(arrows)* in association with nodularity and tiny erosions **(B)**, distal narrowing with a Barrett ulcer *(arrow)* **(C)**, and more severe Barrett stricture *(arrow)* with prestenotic dilation **(D** and **E)**, Single-contrast esophagram demonstrates a short stricture *(arrow)* of the more proximal esophagus, also representing a Barrett stricture.

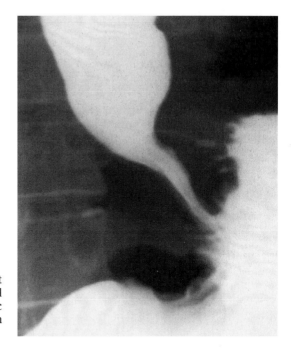

Figure 3–19. Fundoplication. Single-contrast esophagram displays narrowing of the distal esophagus secondary to wrapping of the gastric fundus around the distal esophagus from a Nissen fundoplication.

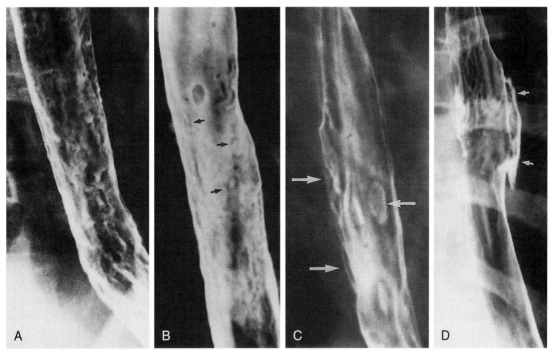

Figure 3–20. Infectious esophagitides. Double-contrast esophagrams reveal findings of the common infectious esophagitides: irregular ragged mucosa of esophageal candidiasis **(A)**, multiple small erosions with lucent rims of surrounding edema *(arrows)* from herpetic esophagitis **(B)**, large ulcers with surrounding halos of edema *(arrows)* from cytomegalovirus esophagitis **(C)**, and a large flat human immunodeficiency virus ulcer *(arrows)* **(D)**.

mal esophagus near the aortic arch or left main stem bronchus impressions (Fig. 3–21). Antibiotics are the most common offending agent, particularly doxycycline and tetracycline, but other drugs include potassium chloride, aspirin, and quinidine.

Caustic esophagitis is caused by ingestion of caustic chemicals and results in immediate sloughing of the mucosa, inflammation, and eventual stricture formation that can be focal or extend over long segments (Fig. 3–22). Common agents include drain cleaner (lye) and other household cleaners. These agents commonly are ingested accidentally by children or deliberately by adults as a suicide attempt.

Other less common esophagitides include Crohn disease, Behçet disease, epidermolysis bullosa, pemphigoid, and graft-versus-host disease. Inflammation and strictures of the esophagus may occur from long-term nasogastric intubation and irradiation of mediastinal or lung tumors.

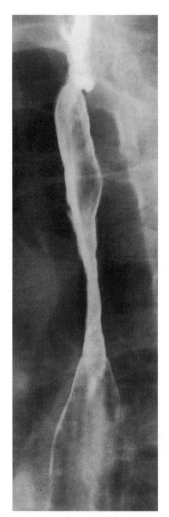

Figure 3–22. Lye stricture. Double-contrast esophagram shows a long stricture of the mid-esophagus resulting from lye ingestion.

Benign Neoplasms

Benign esophageal tumors of the esophagus are uncommon but not rare, accounting for nearly 20% of esophageal neoplasms. The following lesions constitute most benign esophageal masses: leiomyoma, fibrovascular polyp, cysts, squamous papilloma, fibroma, hemangioma, lipoma, and adenoma.

Accounting for nearly half of benign esophageal neoplasms, the **leiomyoma** produces a defect in the wall of the esophagus with right or slightly obtuse angles at its margin, indicating an intramural location. Fatty attenuation tissue can be seen in lipomas on CT scan. **Leiomyomas** often are asymptomatic but can be large enough to cause dysphagia (Fig. 3–23).

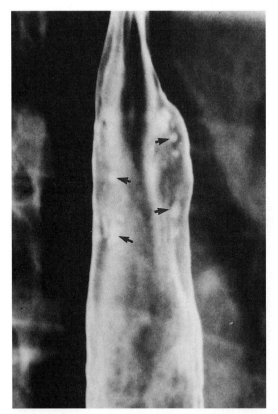

Figure 3–21. Chemical erosions. Double-contrast esophagram of the proximal esophagus illustrates multiple rounded collections of barium *(arrows)* representing erosions from aspirin ingestion.

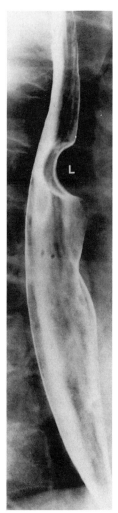

Figure 3–23. Esophageal leiomyoma. Double-contrast esophagram shows an intramural defect representing an esophageal leiomyoma (L).

Congenital **duplication cysts** and **retention cysts** appear as intramural lesions. These cysts cannot be differentiated other than by CT or endoscopic ultrasound, which can determine their cystic nature.

The **fibrovascular polyp** is often a large bulky tumor with a pedicle that originates in the proximal esophagus and sometimes in the hypopharynx. The tumor often widens the esophageal lumen. It is thought that these mesenchymal tumors elongate and form pedicles as a consequence of prolonged exposure to the forces of peristalsis (Fig. 3–24).

Squamous papilloma tends to be a single, small, smooth nodule that measures several millimeters in diameter. Papillomas may be

multiple and on occasion diffusely involve the esophagus.

Malignant Neoplasms

Squamous cell carcinoma and adenocarcinoma are the two most prevalent malignancies of the esophagus. **Squamous cell carcinoma** has multiple different radiographic appearances (Fig. 3–25). Early tumors often are manifested by small protruding masses, plaquelike lesions, or small polyps. More advanced carcinomas usually can be grouped into four major classifications: infiltrating, polypoid, ulcerative, and varicoid. Predisposing factors include head and neck tumors, achalasia, chemical strictures, Plummer-Vinson syndrome, radiation, and celiac disease. The major risk factors in the United States are alcohol and tobacco use, which

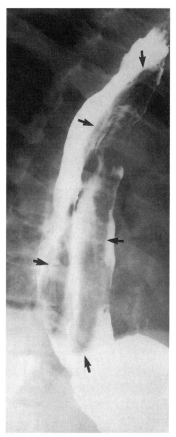

Figure 3–24. Fibrovascular polyp. Single-contrast esophagram reveals an elongated fibrovascular polyp *(arrows)*, occupying most of the esophagus. The patient reportedly would occasionally regurgitate and swallow this pedunculated polyp.

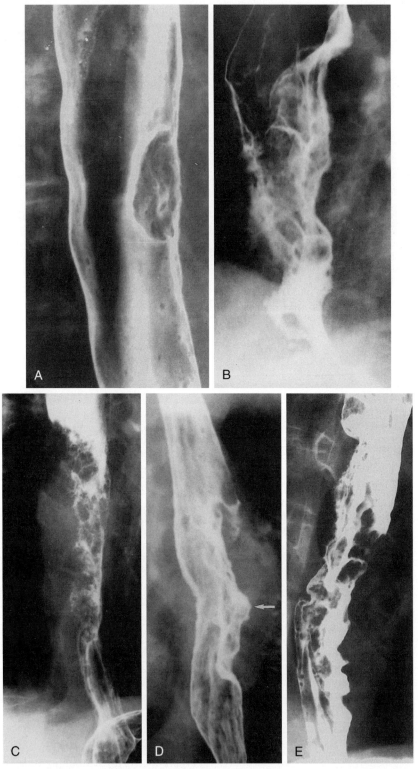

Figure 3–25. Squamous cell carcinoma. Five esophagrams exhibit the varied appearances of squamous cell carcinoma: plaquelike (with small central ulceration) **(A)**, infiltrating **(B)**, polypoid **(C)**, ulcerative (with central ulceration) *(arrow)* **(D)**, and varicoid **(E)**.

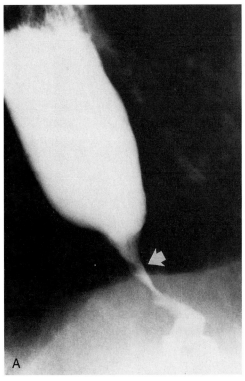

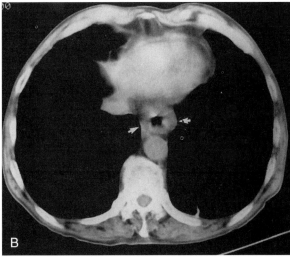

Figure 3–26. Adenocarcinoma. Smooth narrowing of the esophageal wall *(arrows)* is evident in a patient with adenocarcinoma of the distal esophagus on a single-contrast esophagram **(A)** and chest CT scan **(B)**.

are synergistic. Dramatically increased incidences, in geographic areas such as China, are believed to be caused by environmental carcinogens and nutritional deficiencies.

Adenocarcinoma of the esophagus can secondarily originate in the proximal stomach and ascend, causing a nodular constrictive appearance of the distal esophagus (Fig. 3–26). Most primary esophageal adenocarcinomas arise from Barrett mucosa. Similar to squamous cell carcinomas, adenocarcinomas can have a variety of appearances, including plaquelike, polypoid, nodular, infiltrating, ulcerative, and varicoid.

Lymphoma and **Kaposi sarcoma** are radiographically indistinguishable from each other and sometimes from adenocarcinoma. Lymphomatous involvement of the esophagus often arises from outside the esophagus, such as from mediastinal lymph nodes or the stomach. Kaposi sarcoma previously was a rare malignancy, but it now is seen with increasing frequency because of AIDS.

Spindle-cell carcinoma (previously known as *carcinosarcoma*, *pseudosarcoma*, and *polypoid carcinoma*) tends to be large and bulky and causes expansion of the esophageal lumen. It may be indistinguishable from a giant fibrovascular polyp or leiomyosarcoma. **Leiomyosarcoma** is a large bulky lesion that may ulcerate and causes esophageal lumen expansion.

Metastases to the esophagus commonly originate from carcinomas of the stomach, lung, breast, pancreas, and other distant sites. Because of lack of a serosa, esophageal malignancies are likely to invade adjacent structures. A well-known complication of esophageal carcinoma is fistula formation to the tracheobronchial tree. These tumors also metastasize through lymphatic and hematogenous routes.

Miscellaneous Conditions

Esophageal varices are collateral veins that dilate in response to impeded venous flow, usually because of portal hypertension from cirrhosis and less commonly from superior vena cava obstruction. These varices are of great clinical significance because of their tendency to rupture and produce massive hemorrhage. Radiographically, varices present as serpiginous filling defects, which sometimes can be seen only transiently secondary to peristalsis and respiration (Fig. 3–27).

Esophageal foreign bodies in children are represented mostly by lodged coins, toys, and other foreign objects, whereas in adults they comprise mainly impacted food items, such as meat or bones (Fig. 3–28). Most esophageal foreign bodies pass spontaneously, but some require medical intervention. Complications include mural edema, erosion, perforation, and abscess formation.

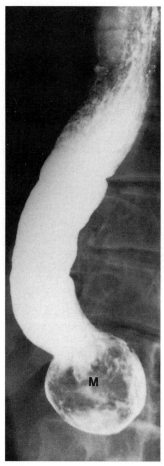

Figure 3–28. Food impaction. Single-contrast esophagram indicates obstruction of the distal esophagus by a filling defect representing lodged meat (M).

The presence of a lodged foreign body in an adult raises suspicion for an instigating esophageal stricture.

Boerhaave syndrome refers to spontaneous perforation of the esophagus that results from a sudden large increase in intraluminal pressure, such as from vomiting, retching, coughing, and blunt trauma. The site of perforation is commonly in the left posterolateral wall of the distal esophagus, just proximal to the gastroesophageal junction, because of the lack of supporting adjacent mediastinal structures. Radiographic findings include pneumomediastinum, subcutaneous emphysema, pleural fluid, and pneumothorax (Fig. 3–29).

Multiple ingenious surgical procedures have been developed to bypass a diseased

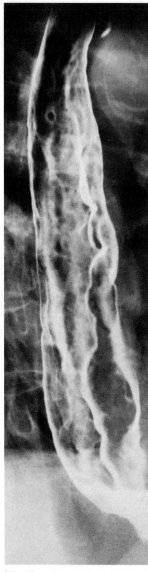

Figure 3–27. Esophageal varices. Double-contrast esophagram reveals large serpiginous filling defects in the midesophagus and distal esophagus from esophageal varices.

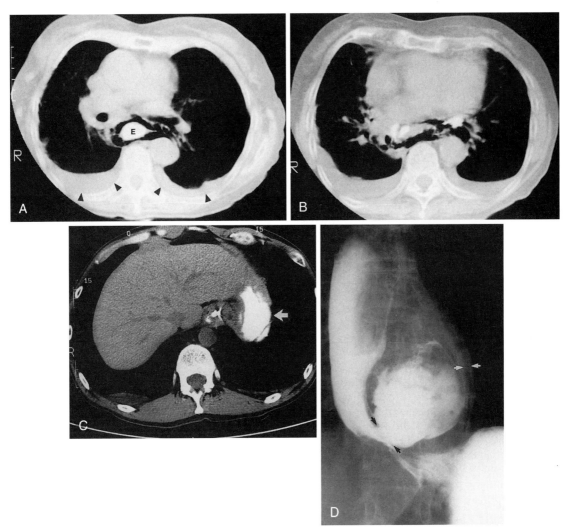

Figure 3–29. Boerhaave syndrome. Representative axial CT sections **(A–C)** through the distal thorax reveal contrast within the esophagus (E), which is surrounded by mediastinal air in a patient with Boerhaave syndrome. Bilateral pleural fluid collections are present *(arrowheads)*. A large extraluminal collection of contrast material is identified inferiorly *(arrow)*. **D,** Water-soluble esophagram reveals the site of esophageal rupture *(black arrows)* as well as pneumomediastinum *(white arrows)*.

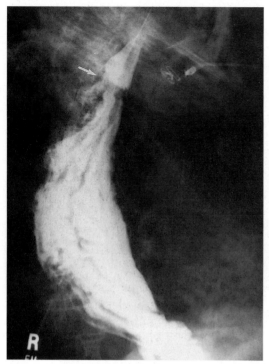

Figure 3–30. Gastric pull-through. Single-contrast barium examination of a gastric pull-through demonstrates the esophagogastric anastomosis *(arrow)*, with most of the stomach pulled up into the chest.

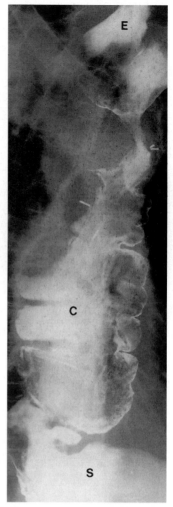

Figure 3–31. Colonic interposition. Single-contrast examination of a colonic interposition indicates the interposed colonic segment (C) spanning the esophageal remnant (E) and stomach (S).

segment of the esophagus. The two most commonly seen techniques are the **esophagogastrectomy (gastric pull-through),** in which the stomach is mobilized and anastomosed to the esophageal remanant (Fig. 3–30), and **colonic interposition**, in which a segment of colon is mobilized and placed in either the anterior or middle mediastinum and anastomosed with the stomach (Fig. 3–31).

Suggested Readings

Gore RM, Levine MS, Laufer I: Textbook of Gastrointestinal Radiology, 2nd ed. Philadelphia, WB Saunders, 2000.

Houston JD, Davis M: Fundamentals of Fluoroscopy. Philadelphia, WB Saunders, 2001.

Laufer I, Levine MS, Rubesin SE: Double Contrast Gastrointestinal Radiology, 3rd ed. Philadelphia, WB Saunders, 1999.

Levine MS: Radiology of the Esophagus. Philadelphia, WB Saunders, 1989.

FOUR

Stomach

Michael Davis, M.D., and Jeffrey D. Houston, M.D.

Normal Anatomy

The stomach has a widely variable shape depending on body habitus and degree of distention. It is a generally J-shaped organ that can be divided into the following anatomic components: fundus, cardia, body, and pyloric antrum and canal (Fig. 4–1).

The abdominal esophagus enters the stomach at the cardiac orifice. The **fundus** refers to the subdiaphragmatic portion of the stomach that is superior and to the left of the cardiac orifice, whereas the **cardia** is a histologically defined region immediately surrounding the cardiac orifice. The **body** (corpus) occupies most of the stomach, lying between the fundus and antrum. The **pylorus** is the caudal third of the stomach that consists of the pyloric **antrum** and pyloric canal. It is distinguished histologically by containing pyloric glands and lacking parietal cells. A thickened band of circular muscle surrounding the pyloric canal creates a sphincter that controls the rate of gastric emptying.

The **lesser curvature** is the concave medial border of the stomach, which normally is located on the patient's right. The **greater curvature** is the much longer convex lateral border of the stomach, which normally is situated on the left. The **angular notch** (incisura angularis) is the sharp angulation in the lesser curvature that demarcates the junction of the body and antrum.

The mucosal pattern of the stomach is seen radiographically as gastric rugae and areae gastricae (Fig. 4–2). **Rugae** are mucosal folds often seen in the nondistended stomach. The **areae gastricae** represent the normal reticular mucosal pattern of the stomach, which is most prominent in the antrum and body.

Imaging Modalities

Common indications for radiologic examination of the stomach include epigastric pain, dyspepsia, nausea, vomiting, hematemesis, and abdominal masses. Examination of the stomach can be performed using single-contrast or double-contrast technique and usually is performed as part of an upper gastrointestinal series (upper GI), in which the esophagus, stomach, and duodenum are imaged concurrently. Biphasic examinations often are performed to incorporate the benefits of each technique. Patients are asked to take nothing by mouth for 6 hours before the examination to ensure that the stomach is empty.

In a routine **single-contrast upper gastrointestinal series** (Fig. 4–3), the stomach is

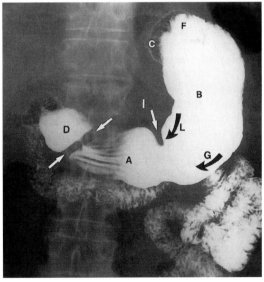

Figure 4–1. Normal anatomy of the stomach. Single-contrast anteroposterior examination allows visualization of the anatomic regions of the stomach: cardia (C), fundus (F), body (B), pyloric antrum (A), pylonic canal *(arrows)*, lesser curvature (L), greater curvature (G), angular notch (incisura angularis) (I). (From Houston JD, Davis M: Fundamentals of Fluoroscopy. Philadelphia, WB Saunders, 2001.)

37

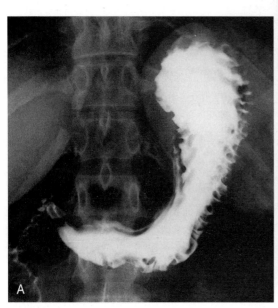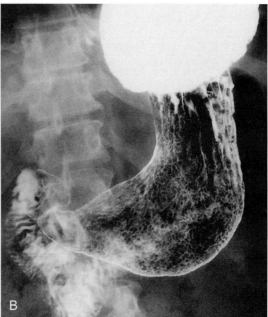

Figure 4–2. Gastric mucosal features. A, Single-contrast examination allows visualization of normal mucosal folds. **B,** Double-contrast examination reveals the finely nodular mucosal pattern of the areae gastricae.

partially filled with a small amount of regular barium (60% weight volume [w/v]). The stomach is compressed, either manually or by using gravity and patient positioning, and each segment is imaged. Additional barium is administered, and images of the filled stomach are obtained. Single-contrast technique allows assessment of the thickness of the gastric folds and estimation of the rate of gastric emptying, but it is not as sensitive as double-contrast technique for detecting small mucosal abnormalities.

In a routine **double-contrast upper gastrointestinal series** (Fig. 4–4), the stomach is paralyzed temporarily with systemically administered glucagon, filled with several ounces of dense barium (200% to 250% w/v), and distended with gas using effervescent granules. Images are obtained as the patient rolls into various positions to coat the mucosa with dense barium.

The **scintigraphic gastric emptying study** is the preferred method of quantifying the rate of gastric emptying. Radiolabeled food substances, such as technetium 99m–sulfur colloid in scrambled eggs or milk, is ingested while sequential images are obtained with a gamma camera, and a time-activity curve is generated. Normally, half of the activity is emptied from the stomach in 90 minutes for solids and 40 minutes for liquids.

Computed tomography (CT) of the stomach has limited applications and is reserved best for further evaluation of already established abnormalities, such as for assessing extramural extension of malignancy. Imaging can be optimized by filling the stomach with dilute contrast immediately before scanning.

Ultrasonography is employed in the diagnosis of hypertrophic pyloric stenosis in neonates. The utility of ultrasound otherwise is limited by intraluminal air.

Functional Abnormalities

Gastroparesis is one of the most common functional abnormalities of the stomach. Seen in conditions such as diabetes and progressive systemic sclerosis, gastroparesis is a disorder of gastric peristalsis. Decreased peristalsis results in functional obstruction, with retention of food particles and fluid, and ensuing gastric dilation (Fig. 4–5).

Gastric outlet obstruction can occur from a variety of conditions, which can be either functional or mechanical. **Hypertrophic pyloric stenosis** generally occurs in neonates and is characterized by hypertrophy of the circular muscle of the pylorus. It normally presents in the first 2 to 6 weeks of life with recurrent vomiting. Measurement of the

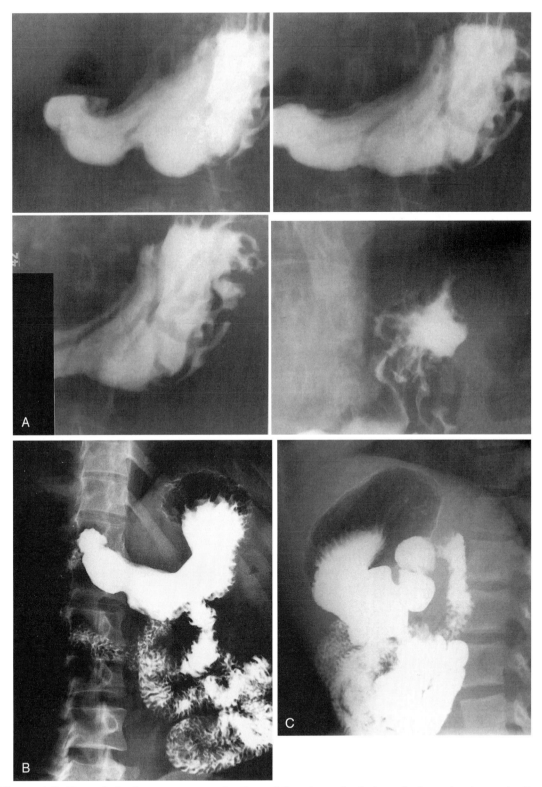

Figure 4–3. Normal single-contrast examination of the stomach. A, In a single-contrast examination, compression films are obtained initially of each gastric segment using only a small amount of barium. After additional barium is ingested, posteroanterior **(B)**, right lateral **(C)**, and sometimes other views of the distended stomach are obtained.

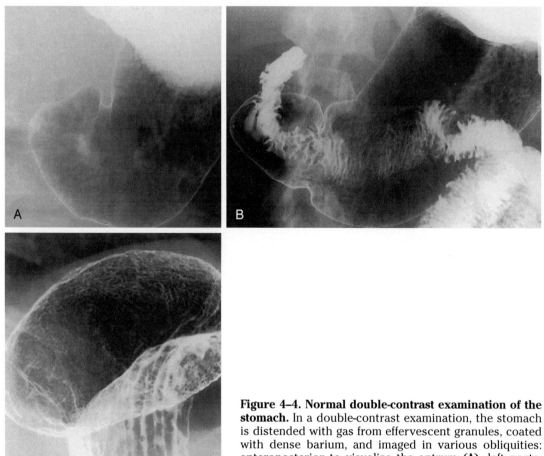

Figure 4–4. Normal double-contrast examination of the stomach. In a double-contrast examination, the stomach is distended with gas from effervescent granules, coated with dense barium, and imaged in various obliquities: anteroposterior to visualize the antrum **(A)**, left posterior oblique to visualize the body **(B)**, and upright to visualize the fundus **(C)**.

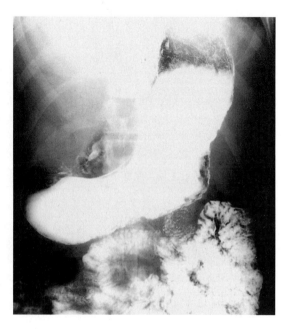

Figure 4–5. Gastric atony. Single-contrast examination shows an enlarged stomach resulting from chronic narcotic abuse.

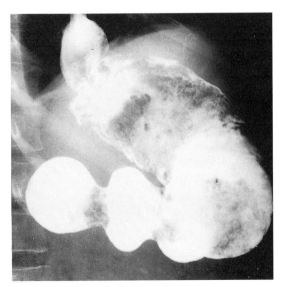

Figure 4–6. Gastric bezoar. Single-contrast examination of the stomach shows distention of the stomach caused by heterogeneous filling defects from gastric bezoars.

pyloric muscle thickness and channel length most often is performed with ultrasound, or a narrowed pyloric channel and a broad muscular shoulder can be documented with barium examination. **Pylorospasm** has a similar clinical presentation as hypertrophic pyloric stenosis but spontaneously disappears after days to weeks.

Gastric **bezoars** are concretions of undigested material sometimes found in the stomach or other parts of the alimentary canal (Fig. 4–6). The major types of bezoars are trichobezoars (hair), phytobezoars (fruit or vegetable fibers), and lactobezoars (milk curd). Gastric surgery and gastroparesis are predisposing conditions for the development of bezoars.

Gastroesophageal reflux refers to regurgitation of gastric contents into the esophagus. It occurs from incompetency of the lower esophageal sphincter, often in association with a hiatal hernia. Mild reflux can occur physiologically in infants but should resolve with development. As discussed previously, refluxed acid can cause significant damage to the esophagus and is associated with mucosal metaplasia and adenocarcinoma formation.

Structural Abnormalities

Rare congenital abnormalities include agastria, microgastria, and gastric duplica-

tion. More common structural abnormalities of the stomach include abnormal position, herniation, diverticula, aberrant rests of pancreatic tissue, webs, duplication cysts, and extrinsic deformity.

Abnormal positioning of the stomach can be due to variant gastric anatomy, dextrogastria, or herniation. **Cascade stomach** is a characteristic variation in gastric configuration that is usually of no clinical significance, in which the fundus lies posteroinferior to the body instead of in its normal, more superior location. When the patient is upright, ingested barium initially accumulates in the posteriorly located fundus, then cascades into the body.

Dextrogastria is a rare condition in which the stomach is located in the right upper quadrant of the abdomen and can be an isolated finding, resulting from complete transposition, or associated with the heterotaxy syndromes, such as asplenia and polysplenia.

Gastric herniations include sliding and paraesophageal hiatal hernias as well as congenital and traumatic diaphragmatic hernias. As previously discussed, the most common hiatal hernia is the sliding type. Hiatal hernias can be large, with much of the stomach located in the chest, and occasionally can be seen on chest radiographs (Fig. 4–7). Paraesophageal and traumatic diaphragmatic hernias can be particularly serious conditions because of the risk of incarceration and strangulation.

Gastric volvulus is a relatively rare condition that can occur at any age. Although volvulus can occur when the stomach is located normally in the abdomen, it is associated most commonly with gastric herniation. The stomach can rotate along its normal long axis (organoaxial volvulus) (Fig. 4–8) or perpendicular to the long axis along the plane of mesenteric attachment of the omentum (mesenteroaxial volvulus).

Gastric diverticula are generally asymptomatic and identified incidentally. Most occur in the posteromedial fundus (Fig. 4–9), with most of the remainder arising along the distal greater curvature. Aberrant **rests of pancreatic tissue** are found commonly in the stomach, particularly in the antrum or in gastric diverticula. They usually present as solitary small, rounded filling defects and occasionally contain a central dimple that connects to a rudimentary duct.

Thin mucosal **webs** rarely can be encoun-

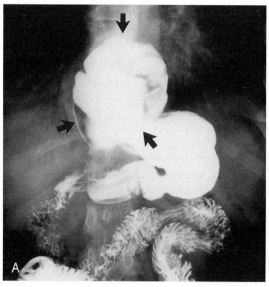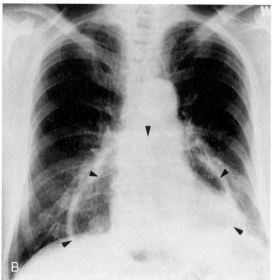

Figure 4–7. Hiatal hernia. A, Single-contrast examination reveals herniation of most of the stomach *(arrows)* into the chest through the esophageal hiatus. **B,** A large rounded lucency *(arrowheads)* is seen projecting over the heart on a posteroanterior chest radiograph in another patient with a large hiatal hernia.

tered in the stomach, usually just proximal to the pylorus. Gastric **duplication cysts** are developmental cystlike structures that are lined by gastric mucosa and contain fluid. They often are located in the distal stomach,

are contiguous with the gastric wall, and can be intramural or extrinsic.

Because of the pliability of the stomach, various adjacent structures easily can produce mass effect on the stomach. Conditions that can result in **extrinsic deformity** include pancreatic masses (e.g., pancreatitis, pseudocysts, neoplasms, and abscesses),

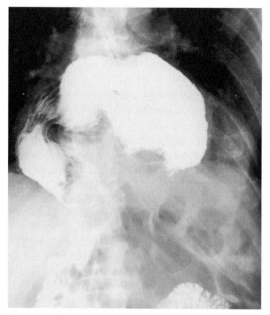

Figure 4–8. Gastric volvulus. Single-contrast examination displays total intrathoracic herniation of the stomach with organoaxial volvulus. Note the inversion of the greater curvature.

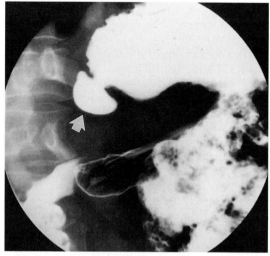

Figure 4–9. Gastric diverticulum. Single-contrast examination illustrates a diverticulum *(arrow)* arising from the medial aspect of the gastric fundus. This is the most common site of gastric diverticula.

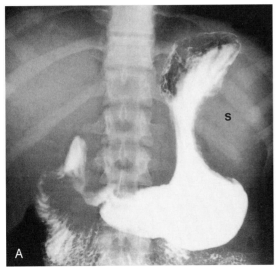 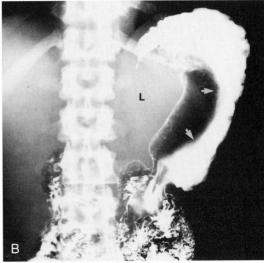

Figure 4–10. Extrinsic gastric impressions. Upper gastrointestinal series reveals abnormal extrinsic mass effect on the stomach caused by splenomegaly (S), displacing the fundus medially **(A)**; and hepatomegaly **(B),** with the enlarged left lobe of the liver (L) displacing the gastric barium column laterally *(arrows).*

abdominal aortic aneurysms, periaortic lymphadenopathy, adrenal masses, splenomegaly, hepatomegaly, and fluid collections in the lesser sac (Fig. 4–10).

Gastritis

Gastritis refers to inflammation of the gastric mucosa, which can result from many causes. Perhaps as a result of lack of consensus regarding a classification scheme, gastritis often is divided simply into acute and chronic categories.

Acute gastritis is a transient process characterized by neutrophilic infiltration. It is associated with nonsteroidal anti-inflammatory drugs (particularly aspirin), alcoholism, heavy smoking, chemotherapy, uremia, systemic infections, severe physical stress (e.g., burns, trauma, surgery), caustic chemical ingestion, irradiation, or mechanical trauma.

Radiographically, acute gastritis appears as an alteration of the mucosal pattern. An **erosion** is a focal loss of superficial epithelium, which creates a defect in the mucosa that does not cross the muscularis mucosa. Hemorrhage may occur and result in massive hematemesis, particularly in alcoholics. **Erosive gastritis** usually is manifested radiographically by small collections of barium surrounded by radiolucent halos that are formed by small mounds of edema. Double-contrast technique is best for showing these

small lesions (Fig. 4–11). In some instances, the mucosal surface pattern can become irregular and nodular, and there can be associated thickening of the gastric folds. Erosions are most common in the antrum, pyloric canal, and duodenal bulb.

The presence of gas in the stomach wall is referred to as **emphysematous gastritis**. Causes of intramural gas include cystic pneumatosis, noninfective interstitial emphysema, and gas-forming infections. **Cystic pneumatosis** is a rare benign idiopathic entity that is seen more commonly in the colon and features rounded submucosal bubbles of gas. Other sources of intramural air include peptic ulcer disease, endoscopic injury or biopsy, and trauma. Infectious emphysematous gastritis is a serious condition caused by infection with gas-forming organisms, such as *Clostridium welchii, Escherichia coli,* and *Staphylococcus aureus,* usually following surgery, infarction, severe gastritis, or corrosive ingestion.

Chronic gastritis is distinguished by chronic mucosal inflammation with predominance of lymphocytes or plasma cells. Causes include chronic infection, autoimmune diseases, alcoholism, heavy smoking, granulomatous conditions, irradiation, and mechanical causes. Chronic gastritis can eventually lead to mucosal atrophy and epithelial metaplasia, creating a foundation for neoplasia.

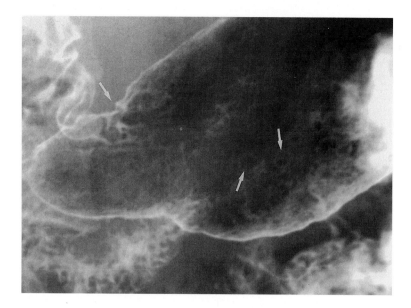

Figure 4–11. Erosive gastritis. Double-contrast technique demonstrates several superficial erosions *(arrows).*

Chronic superficial gastritis refers to limitation of the inflammatory infiltrate to the superficial mucosa and is not visible radiographically. Chronic gastritis may result in coarsened erythematous mucosa, which can be flattened or alternatively boggy-appearing with thickened mucosal folds (Fig. 4–12). With progressive disease, the mucosa becomes thinned and flattened.

Helicobacter pylori, a corkscrew-shaped gram-negative bacterium discovered in 1982, is the cause in most cases of acute and chronic gastritis and the cause of most peptic (gastric and duodenal) ulcers. The bacte-

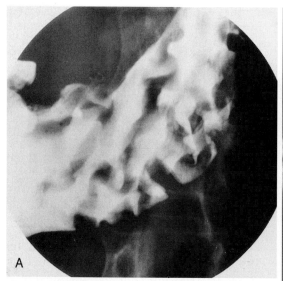
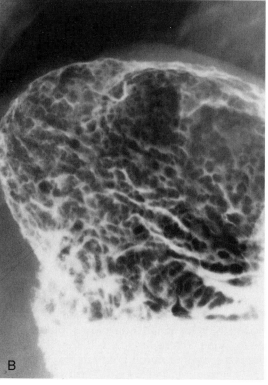

Figure 4–12. Gastritis. A, A spot film from a single-contrast upper gastrointestinal series illustrates enlarged gastric folds in the body of the stomach in a patient with gastritis. **B,** Double-contrast examination of the fundus illustrates multiple filling defects carpeting the fundus, representing enlarged areae gastricae in another patient with gastritis.

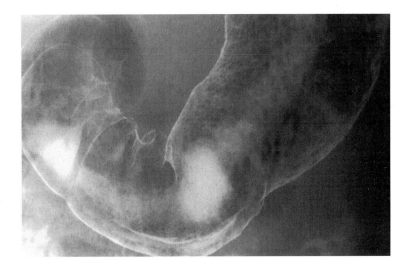

Figure 4–13. Atrophic gastritis. Double-contrast examination reveals loss of the normal mucosal features of the stomach from long-standing atrophic gastritis.

ria live in the gastric mucus layer or adherent to the epithelial lining. Bacterial enzymes destroy the mucus glycoproteins and expose the underlying epithelium to gastric acid. Approximately two thirds of the world's population is infected with this organism. Antral nodularity and narrowing are indicative of *H. pylori* gastritis. Large gastric folds, with or without ulceration or erosions, are the best predictors of *H. pylori* gastritis.

H. pylori predominately causes antral gastritis, whereas autoimmune disease is responsible for predominantly corpus (proximal) gastritis. When active gastritis is determined to be *H. pylori* negative, Crohn disease should be a diagnostic consideration.

Other infectious gastritides include tuberculosis, histoplasmosis, candidiasis, and syphilis. Less common types of gastritis include eosinophilic gastritis and radiation gastritis.

Atrophic gastritis indicates more diffuse inflammation, with thinning of the mucosa and a decreased quantity of gastric glands. In the most severe form, **gastric atrophy**, there is complete loss of the gastric glands, marked mucosal thinning, and intestinal metaplasia of the stomach. The radiographic findings of atrophic gastritis and gastric atrophy include almost complete disappearance of folds in the proximal two thirds of the stomach, a generally tubular appearance of the stomach, small widely spaced areae gastricae, or virtual absence of the areae gastricae (Fig. 4–13).

Corrosive chemical ingestion can cause immediate sloughing of gastric mucosa and severe gastritis. Eventual scarring can create severe narrowing and rigidity of the affected segment (Fig. 4–14).

Peptic Ulcer Disease

Gastric ulcers represent disruptions of the mucosa that extend into or through the

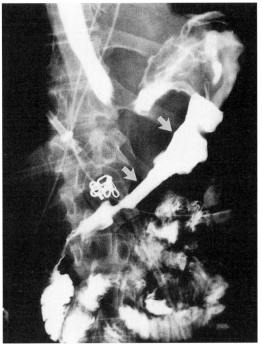

Figure 4–14. Lye stricture. Single-contrast examination displays marked narrowing and distortion of the entire stomach, particularly the gastric body and antrum *(arrows)* resulting from lye ingested in a suicide attempt. Note the narrowing of the proximal duodenum.

submucosa. Ulcers often are remitting and relapsing lesions that can attain large size and perforate the gastric wall. They are found most commonly in middle-aged to older adults. Ulcerogenic factors include *H. pylori* infection, cigarette smoking, alcoholism, drugs (particularly nonsteroidal anti-inflammatory drugs and corticosteroids), severe physical stress (e.g., shock, burns, trauma, surgery, sepsis), and perhaps personality traits.

Benign ulcers account for about 95% of all gastric ulcers. Approximately 90% of malignant ulcers are caused by adenocarcinoma, whereas the remainder are caused by lymphoma and other rare malignancies.

Up to 80% of gastric ulcers are detected with double-contrast barium examinations. Small ulcers can be radiographically unapparent because of small size of the craters, shallowness, or effacement of small craters by gaseous distention. The advantages of increased sensitivity of small ulcer detection with gastroscopy have to be weighed against the more invasive, expensive, and time-consuming disadvantages of endoscopy.

Multiple radiographic criteria can be applied to categorize ulcers as probably benign, probably malignant, or indeterminate (Table 4–1). Characteristics used to categorize ulcers include shape, depth of penetration, appearance of adjacent mucosal folds, appearance of an ulcer collar or mound, and observation of peristalsis (Fig. 4–15).

Most ulcers are seen radiographically en face as collections of barium in the craters. Ulcers most commonly are round but can have linear, irregular, or serpiginous shapes. Benign ulcers are classically round or ovoid (Fig. 4–15*A*), whereas malignant ulcers can have more irregular shapes.

Because ulcers often incite local edema, an **ulcer mound** is a commonly visualized elevation of tissue surrounding the ulcer. Benign ulcer mounds are characteristically smooth and symmetrical surrounding the central umbilication (Fig. 4–15*B*), whereas malignant mounds often are irregular or asymmetrical and have an eccentric crater.

Contraction of collagenous tissue produced at the ulcer base can result in converging mucosal folds that become apparent because of decreased distensibility when the stomach is compressed or distended. Mucosal folds of benign ulcers generally radiate smoothly to the ulcer crater (see Fig. 4–15*A*) or fade into the mound, whereas folds associated with malignant ulcers can be thickened and irregular, may merge before reaching the ulcer, or may not extend to the crater edge.

In profile, barium can be seen protruding into the ulcer cavity. **Penetration** refers to the ulcer crater projecting beyond the gastric lumen. Benign ulcers often protrude beyond the expected normal contour of the stomach (Fig. 4–15*C*), whereas malignant ulcers generally are more shallow.

After destruction of the gastric mucosa, the more susceptible submucosa becomes vulnerable to the gastric acid and enzymes. Rapid destruction of the submucosa leads to **undermining** of the mucosa, which is evidence of benignity. Extension of the ulcer

Table 4–1.
Radiographic Characteristics Associated with Benign and Malignant Ulcers

	Benign	Malignant
Shape	Round, oval, linear	Irregular
Penetration	Ulcer protrudes beyond the expected normal contour of the stomach	Ulcer does not generally protrude beyond the expected normal contour of the stomach
Mucosal folds	Smoothly radiate to the ulcer crater or fade into the mound	Thickened, irregular, may merge before reaching crater, do not extend to crater edge
Collar	Smooth collar across opening	Thick, irregular, or nodular margin
Ulcer mound	Smooth symmetrical mound of edema with central crater	Irregular or asymmetrical mound of edema with eccentric crater
Peristalsis	Normal	Abnormal
Other	Hampton line	Rigidity of adjacent wall, Carman meniscus sign
Healing	Significant healing within 2–3 weeks, with resolution after 6 weeks of medical therapy	Fail to heal completely with medical therapy

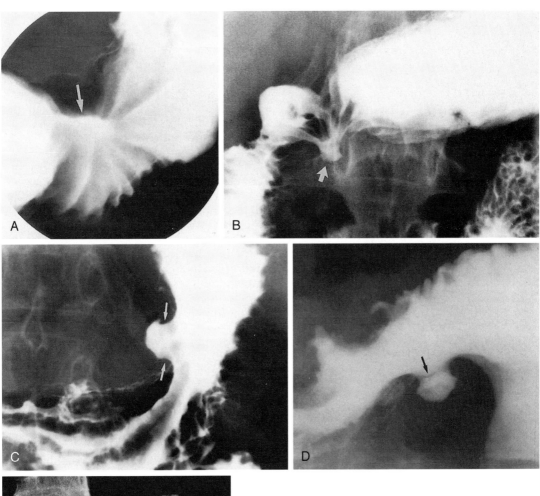

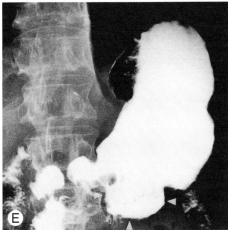

Figure 4–15. Benign gastric ulcers. Single-contrast examinations in multiple patients reveal various radiographic characteristics of benign gastric ulcers: an ovoid posterior wall ulcer *(arrow)* in the body of the stomach with normal-sized gastric folds terminating at the margin of the ulcer crater **(A)**, a distal greater curvature ulcer *(arrow)* with retraction of the gastric folds toward the ulcer bed and a smooth mound of surrounding edema **(B)**, a lesser curvature ulcer with a faintly seen collar *(arrows)* and a crater that protrudes well beyond the lumen of the stomach **(C)**, a Hampton line *(arrow)* **(D)**, and a huge ulcer *(arrowheads)* along the greater curvature of the antrum from excessive aspirin usage **(E)**.

into the submucosa occasionally can be radiographically evident as a **Hampton line,** which is a 1- to 2-mm radiolucent line that traverses the neck of benign ulcers and represents a thin lip of mucosa that overhangs the orifice. This line is a virtually pathognomonic feature of a benign ulcer. The **ulcer collar** is seen more commonly and refers to a radiolucent rim seen in necks of deep ulcers, representing enema and undermining of the mucosa (Fig. 4–15D). Benign collars are often smooth, as opposed to thick, irregular, or nodular collars of malignant ulcers. A **collar-button** shape can result from un-

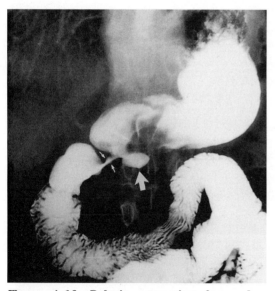

Figure 4–16. Pyloric narrowing from ulcer edema. Single-contrast examination illustrates a benign ulcer in the distal antrum *(large arrow)* along the greater curvature with radiating mucosal folds. A pyloric channel stricture *(small arrows)* is present just distal to the ulcer.

not all, patients with de novo ulcer formation should proceed to endoscopic biopsy to exclude a neoplastic cause. Regardless of the initial radiographic appearance, posttreatment follow-up of peptic ulcer disease is recommended to assess for resolution.

The size, location, and number of ulcers are not reliable signs of malignancy. Ulcers can become quite large. Benign gastric ulcers in the gastric fundus are rare.

The main complications of peptic ulceration are bleeding, obstruction, perforation, and scarring. During active bleeding, a filling defect in the ulcer crater may be seen that represents a blood clot. Obstruction occurs in less than 5% of cases of peptic ulcer disease. Obstructions are caused by scarring and stenosis near the pylorus or significant inflammatory reaction around an active ulcer at the pylorus (Fig. 4–16). Scarring can result in permanent distortion of the gastric folds (Fig. 4–17). Ulceration through the serosa occurs in 5% to 11% of cases, with perforation into the peritoneal cavity or adjacent organs.

dermining, which makes the base of the ulcer appear wider than the orifice.

All patients with active gastritis or peptic ulcer disease should be tested for *H. pylori* infection. Documentation of infection can be obtained with IgG serology, urea breath test, or biopsy. Treatment regimens generally include antibiotics in conjunction with an H_2 blocker or proton-pump inhibitor. Most, if

Hypertrophic Gastropathy

Hypertrophic gastropathy encompasses a group of rare conditions that are characterized by marked thickening of the gastric folds. These diseases are not caused primarily by inflammation, but rather by hyperplasia.

Ménétrier disease is an idiopathic condi-

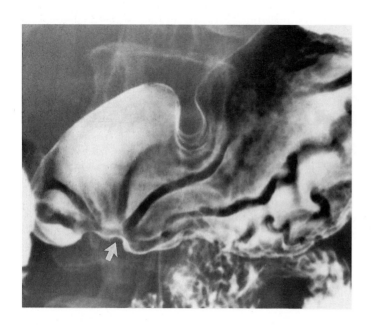

Figure 4–17. Gastric ulcer scar. Double-contrast examination displays an ulcer scar *(arrow)* along the greater curvature of the distal stomach with gastric folds abruptly terminating at the scar.

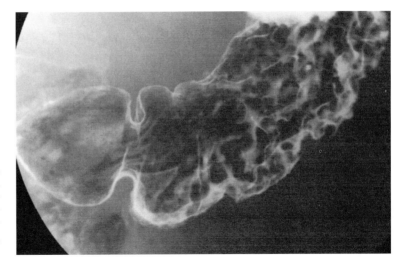

Figure 4–18. Ménétrier disease. Double-contrast examination reveals markedly thickened folds in the body of the stomach, with poor mucosal coating with barium from hypersecretion.

tion that typically occurs in middle-aged men. It is seen radiographically as massive enlargement of gastric rugal folds owing to hyperplasia and hypertrophy of gastric glands (Fig. 4–18). This condition is seen predominantly in the gastric body, usually with lesser involvement of the fundus and sparing of the antrum. Hypochlorhydria is caused by loss of parietal cells. Excessive mucus secretion can cause systemic protein loss (protein-losing gastroenteropathy) and create whirled patterns of mucus within the barium that are characteristic of this disease. There is a known association with carcinoma of the stomach and a strong association with cytomegalovirus in children.

Zollinger-Ellison syndrome is composed of the triad of an islet cell tumor (gastrinoma), gastric hypersecretion, and recalcitrant peptic ulcer disease. Radiographically, Zollinger-Ellison syndrome presents as markedly enlarged folds in the stomach, duodenum, and jejunum with multiple ulcer-

ations and dilation of the proximal small bowel. Gastrin-secreting islet cell tumors of the pancreas are responsible in 90% of cases, and ectopic gastrinomas, usually in the duodenum, are responsible in the remaining 10% of cases. Other causes of thickened gastric folds include gastritis, lymphoma, Kaposi sarcoma, varices, amyloidosis, and Crohn disease.

Benign Neoplasms

Benign gastric neoplasms include tumors of mucosal and mesenchymal origin. Mucosal neoplasms often are manifested as polyps. Two major categories of benign **gastric polyps** exist: hyperplastic polyps and adenomatous polyps.

Hyperplastic polyps are smooth ovoid lesions that are generally sessile and smaller than 1 cm (Fig. 4–19). They have no malig-

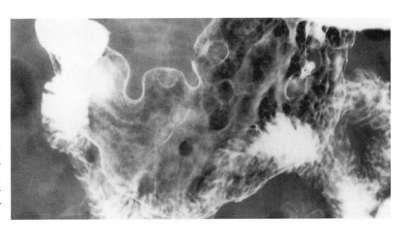

Figure 4–19. Hyperplastic gastric polyps. Double-contrast examination exhibits multiple round defects scattered throughout the stomach.

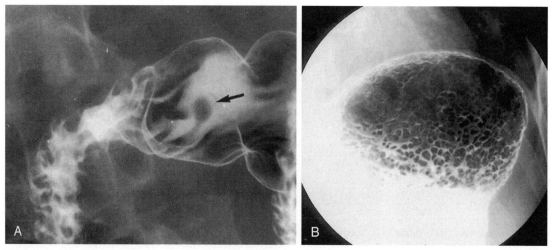

Figure 4–20. Gastric polyps. A, Double-contrast examination shows a solitary filling defect in the antrum *(arrow)*, which was proved to be an adenomatous polyp. **B,** Double-contrast examination shows carpeting of the gastric fundus with fundic gland (hamartomatous) polyps in a patient with Gardner syndrome.

nant potential and are seen most frequently in the setting of chronic gastritis.

Adenomatous polyps are typically larger than 1 cm and infrequently may degenerate into gastric adenocarcinoma and are removed endoscopically on discovery. They often are single and may be sessile or pedunculated (Fig. 4–20). Polyps occasionally reach 3 to 4 cm in diameter before detection.

Submucosal gastric lesions are made up mostly of mesenchymal tissue and are asymptomatic, although the most common smooth muscle tumor of the stomach, the

leiomyoma (Fig. 4–21), has been known to ulcerate and bleed. Most of these tumors are indistinguishable radiographically.

Malignant Neoplasms

Gastric adenocarcinoma is the most common malignancy of the stomach. Risk factors include diet, adenomatous polyps, pernicious anemia, partial gastrectomy, and chronic atrophic gastritis. Gastric carcinomas can have various appearances (Fig. 4–22), which can be grouped based on the

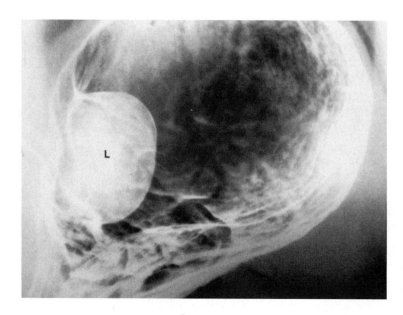

Figure 4–21. Gastric leiomyoma. Double-contrast examination of the proximal stomach shows smooth filling defect involving the medial wall of the fundus, representing a leiomyoma (L) of the stomach. This is a common site of gastric leiomyomas.

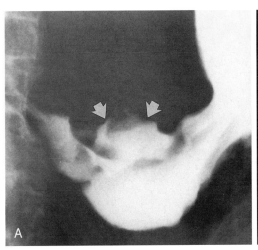 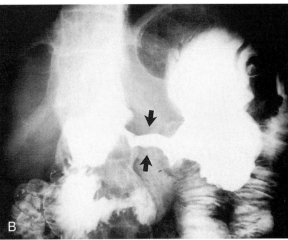

Figure 4–22. Gastric adenocarcinoma. Single-contrast examinations demonstrate an irregular ulceration *(arrows)* along the lesser curvature of the antrum from an adenocarcinoma (Carman meniscus sign) **(A)** and a circumferential infiltrating adenocarcinoma involving the distal stomach, particularly the distal antrum *(arrows)* **(B).**

macroscopic growth pattern: exophytic masses, flat or depressed superficial lesions, infiltrating tumors, and excavated ulcers.

Exophytic tumors generally present as irregular intraluminal polypoid masses. Superficial lesions can show mucosal irregularity, gastric wall rigidity, mucosal flattening with a definite margin, and mucosal nodularity. Gastric carcinoma may present as an ulcerated mass or as an ulceration without a definite mass.

The **Carman meniscus sign** is a sign of malignancy that occurs when an ulcerated neoplasm straddles the lesser curvature of the stomach. The sign is created by apposition of the periphery of the two halves of the ulcer creating a semicircular filling defect outlining trapped barium in the central ulceration that assumes a meniscus shape (Fig. 4–22A).

The pathogenesis of **gastric lymphoma** often begins with accumulation of mucosa-associated lymphoid tissue (MALT) in response to infection of the stomach by *H. pylori*. Rarely, this lymphoid infiltrate contains cells with a growth advantage. Ultimately a low-grade gastric lymphoma results, but it may regress completely after eradication of *H. pylori* from the patient's stomach. If the infection is not eradicated, the low-grade lymphoma ultimately may undergo high-grade transformation.

The radiographic appearance of lymphoma usually is of two types: the infiltrating form, with segmentally or diffusely enlarged polypoid or nodular folds that may ulcerate, and the ulcerating type in which the polypoid or nodular folds are ulcerated.

The incidence of **Kaposi sarcoma** has increased with the acquired immunodeficiency syndrome (AIDS) epidemic. Kaposi sarcoma can present as an ulcerative lesion or can mimic infiltrating lymphoma or severe gastritis, with enlarged and irregular gastric folds (Fig. 4–23).

When a **malignant gastric ulcer** is encountered radiographically, the differential diagnosis includes adenocarcinoma, leiomyosarcoma, lymphoma, Kaposi sarcoma, and metastatic disease. Ulcerating gastric lymphomas and metastases can create a target appearance that is formed by a central barium collection surrounded by a sharply circumscribed tumor mass (Fig. 4–24). Multiple ulcerating lesions in the stomach sometimes are referred to as *bull's eye* or **target lesions**. The most common cause of multiple target lesions is metastatic disease, particularly including breast, lung, and pancreatic cancers as well as melanoma.

Miscellaneous Conditions

Similar to esophageal varices, **gastric varices** are collateral veins that dilate in response to impeded venous flow, usually because of portal hypertension. Radiographically, gastric varices present as thickened serpiginous folds in the region of the gastro-

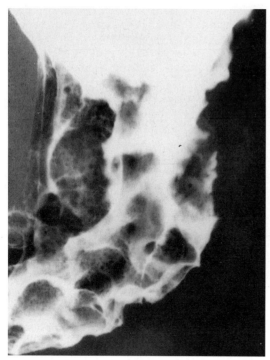

Figure 4–23. Kaposi sarcoma. Single-contrast examination illustrates markedly enlarged and irregular gastric folds throughout the distal body and antrum in a patient with advanced Kaposi sarcoma.

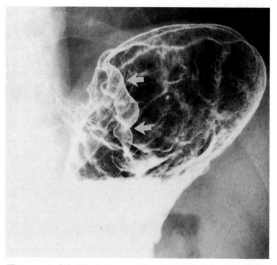

Figure 4–25. Gastric varices. Double-contrast examination of the fundus shows thickened serpiginous folds representing gastric varices *(arrows)*.

esophageal junction, fundus, or proximal body (Fig. 4–25). Varices often can assume a rounded grapelike appearance.

Several types of gastric surgery are commonly encountered radiologically: fundoplication, gastrectomy, pyloroplasty, and gastric plication (Fig. 4–26). As discussed

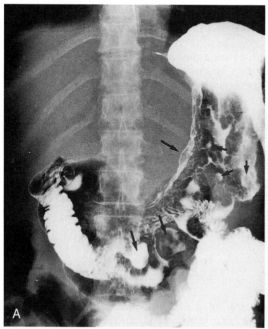

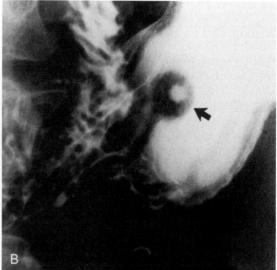

Figure 4–24. Metastatic disease of the stomach. Single-contrast examinations display diffuse infiltration, with grossly thickened folds and ulcerations *(arrows)* throughout the stomach from metastatic breast carcinoma **(A),** and a rounded filling defect *(arrow)* with a central ulceration (target lesion) from metastatic lung carcinoma **(B).**

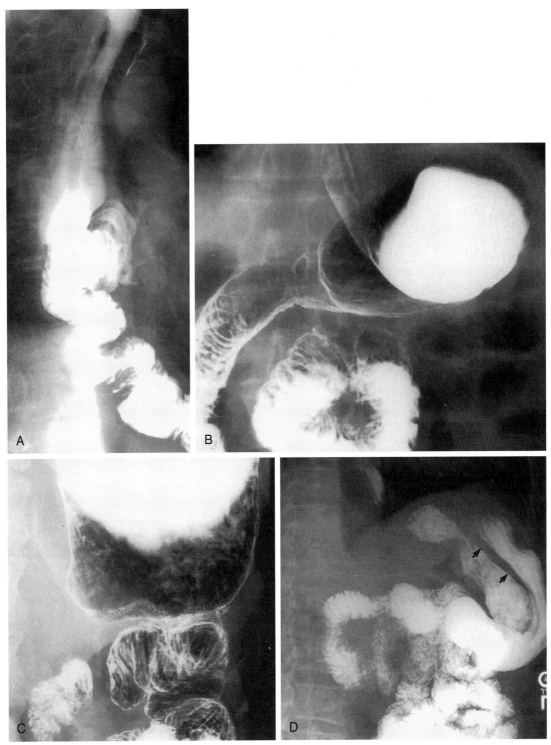

Figure 4–26. Postoperative stomach. Total gastrectomy with esophagojejunostomy **(A),** Billroth I partial gastrectomy with gastroduodenostomy **(B),** Billroth II partial gastrectomy with gastrojejunostomy **(C),** and vertical gastric banding *(arrows)* **(D).**

previously, the various **gastric fundoplication** procedures involve hiatal hernia reduction, restoration of the abdominal segment of the esophagus, and wrapping varying degrees of the gastric fundus around the distal esophagus to hinder gastroesophageal reflux (see Fig. 3–19).

To maintain continuity of the alimentary tract, an **esophagojejunostomy** can be performed after a total gastrectomy. Partial gastrectomies can be performed to resect a diseased segment of the stomach. Of the many eponymic variations, the Billroth procedures are the most widely known. The **Billroth I** consists of partial gastrectomy with gastroduodenostomy, whereas the **Billroth II** consists of partial gastrectomy with gastrojejunostomy.

A **pyloroplasty** is a procedure that widens the pyloric channel to promote gastric emptying. **Gastric plication**, such as the vertical gastric banding procedure, involves dividing the lumen to create a smaller pouch to promote weight loss.

Suggested Readings

Gore RM, Levine MS, Laufer I: Textbook of Gastrointestinal Radiology, 2nd ed. Philadelphia, WB Saunders, 2000.

Houston JD, Davis M: Fundamentals of Fluoroscopy. Philadelphia, WB Saunders, 2001.

Laufer I, Levine MS, Rubesin SE: Double Contrast Gastrointestinal Radiology, 3rd ed. Philadelphia, WB Saunders, 1999.

Marshak RH, Lindner AE, Maklansky D: Radiology of the Stomach. Philadelphia, WB Saunders, 1983.

FIVE

Duodenum

Jeffrey D. Houston, M.D., and Michael Davis, M.D.

Normal Anatomy

The duodenum is characteristically C-shaped and extends from the gastric pylorus to the ligament of Treitz. The duodenum is divided into four numbered anatomic segments (Fig. 5–1). The first or **superior portion** of the duodenum contains the **duodenal bulb** and extends superolaterally from the pylorus. In contrast to the remainder of the duodenum, which is retroperitoneal, the proximal several centimeters of this segment are intraperitoneal and freely movable. Behind the duodenal bulb lies the common bile duct, gastroduodenal artery, and portal vein. An impression from the common bile duct occasionally can be seen radiographically (Fig. 5–2*A*). The gallbladder abuts the proximal duodenum anterolaterally and occasionally casts an impression on the duodenum (Fig. 5–2*B*).

The second or **descending portion** courses lateral to the spine and contains the major and minor papillae, which represent the orifices of the main and accessory pancreatic ducts. The third or **horizontal portion** crosses transversely to the left, anterior to the superior vena cava, aorta, and spine. The superior mesenteric vessels cross this segment anteriorly in a craniocaudad fashion. The fourth or **ascending portion** ascends to the left of the aorta and terminates at the duodenojejunal flexure. The duodenojejunal flexure is supported by the ligament of Treitz, which classically is located at the level of the left L1 pedicle.

The duodenal bulb has characteristically smooth mucosal features (Fig. 5–3), whereas the remainder of the duodenum contains folds of mucosa, known as the **circular folds** of Kerkring. The second and third portions of the duodenum are molded around the head of the pancreas. The submucosa of the duodenum contains tubular **glands of Brunner**, which deliver succus entericus (mucous secretions) into the crypts of Lieberkühn in the intervillar spaces.

Imaging Modalities

Common indications for radiologic examination of the duodenum include epigastric pain, vomiting, hematemesis, and abdominal masses. Similar to the stomach, examination of the duodenum can be performed using single-contrast or double-contrast technique (Fig. 5–4) and usually is performed as part of an upper gastrointestinal series. Biphasic examinations often are performed to incor-

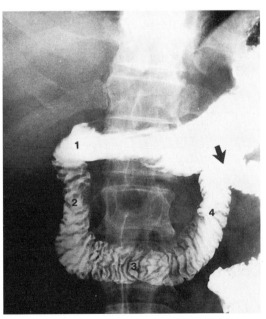

Figure 5–1. Normal anatomy of the duodenum. Single-contrast gastrointestinal series illustrates the anatomic segments of the duodenum: superior (1), descending (2), horizontal (3), and ascending (4). The ligament of Treitz inserts at the duodenojejunal junction *(arrow).*

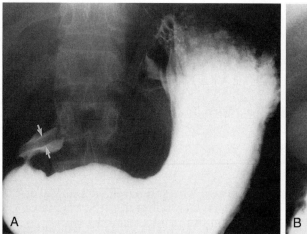
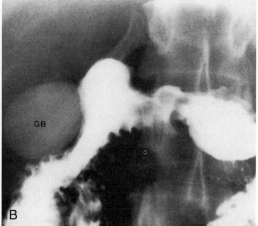

Figure 5–2. Normal extrinsic deformities of the duodenum. Single-contrast examinations reveal extrinsic compression of the duodenum by normal structures: **A,** Common bile duct *(arrows)*. **B,** Gallbladder (GB). Vicarious excretion of iodinated contrast agent allows visualization of the gallbladder.

porate the benefits of each technique. Patients are asked to have nothing by mouth for 6 hours before the examination to ensure that the stomach and duodenum are empty.

In a routine **single-contrast upper gastrointestinal series**, images of the filled duodenum are obtained, with particular attention given to the duodenal bulb. Single-contrast technique allows the assessment of the thickness of the duodenal folds, but is not as sensitive as double-contrast technique for detecting small duodenal abnormalities.

In a routine **double-contrast upper gastrointestinal series**, the gut is paralyzed temporarily with systemically administered gluca-

gon, filled with a small amount of dense barium (200% to 250% weight volume [w/v]), and distended with gas using effervescent granules. Dedicated images of the duodenal bulb are obtained. Double-contrast technique affords superior discrimination of fine mucosal detail.

Computed tomography (CT) of the duodenum has limited applications and often is reserved for further evaluation of already established abnormalities, such as for assessing extrinsic compression. Imaging can be optimized by filling the stomach with dilute barium (1% to 2% w/v) immediately before scanning.

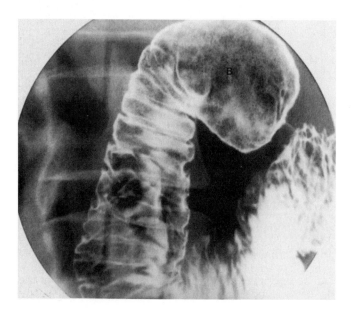

Figure 5–3. Normal duodenal bulb. Double-contrast examination allows visualization of the normal mucosal features of the duodenal bulb (B). The feathery mucosal pattern represents duodenal villi.

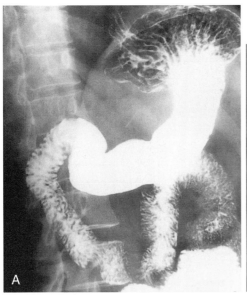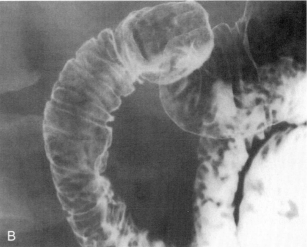

Figure 5–4. Normal duodenal barium examinations. Normal single-contrast **(A)** and double-contrast **(B)** examinations of the duodenum.

Structural Abnormalities

Duodenal atresia results from a complete failure of embryologic recanalization. About one third of the cases of duodenal atresia are associated with Down syndrome. The classic radiographic finding of duodenal atresia is the **"double-bubble" sign**, in which the stomach and proximal duodenum become distended with air that cannot be passed distally (Fig. 5–5).

Duodenal stenosis results from conditions that cause luminal narrowing, such as partial failure of recanalization, webs, encircling

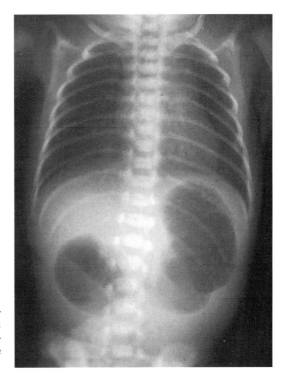

Figure 5–5. Duodenal atresia. Anteroposterior babygram displays the classic "double-bubble" sign of duodenal atresia. The proximal bubble represents gas in the stomach, whereas the distal bubble represents gas in the proximal duodenum.

pancreatic tissue (annular pancreas) (Fig. 5–6), or a preduodenal portal vein. **Superior mesenteric artery syndrome** is another cause of duodenal stenosis that is encountered occasionally, especially in thin individuals. In this condition, there is compression of the duodenum against the aorta by the superior mesenteric artery, resulting in partial or complete obstruction of the duodenum (Fig. 5–7). This abnormality can be precipitated by loss of the normal fat surrounding the superior mesenteric artery.

Duplications of the duodenum are rare and result from abnormal recanalization. Most duplications are cystic, but tubular duplications can occur. A cystic duplication that does not communicate with the lumen is known as a **duodenal duplication cyst**. Large cysts can cause duodenal obstruction.

During normal fetal development, the midgut (precursor of most of the duodenum, small intestine, and right colon) rotates 270 degrees around the origin of the superior mesenteric artery. Most of the duodenum becomes fixed to the posterior abdominal wall, and its mesentery is absorbed. If this process does not progress normally, **malro-**

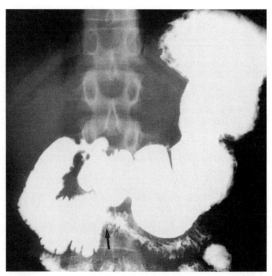

Figure 5–7. Superior mesenteric artery syndrome. Single-contrast examination exhibits partial obstruction of the third portion of the duodenum *(arrow)* with prestenotic dilation, resulting from compression between the superior mesenteric artery and the aorta.

tation occurs. The midgut derivatives assume an abnormal position in the abdomen, and the mesentery lacks normal fixation. The most reliable radiographic indicator of malrotation is an abnormal position of the duodenojejunal junction (Fig. 5–8).

In an attempt to fix the colon to the posterior abdominal wall, the body forms diagonally oriented fibrous bands of peritoneum. These **Ladd bands** can obstruct the duodenum, often the second portion. Twisting of the abnormally shortened small bowel mesentery around the axis of the superior mesenteric artery can produce bowel obstruction and impeded circulation with subsequent infarction. Radiographically, **midgut volvulus** results in obstruction of the third portion of the duodenum, just distal to the ampulla of Vater, and gives a "corkscrew" appearance to the duodenum. Malrotation with volvulus can occur at any age, but generally presents in the first weeks of life with bilious vomiting.

Heterotopic gastric mucosa is an uncommon finding in which islands of gastric mucosa are present, usually in the base of the duodenal bulb, with the islands measuring 1 to 3 mm in diameter and having polygonal shapes. Benign **lymphoid hyperplasia** represents lymphoid follicles measuring 1 to 2 mm that are seen occasionally in the duodenal bulb. Rests of **heterotopic pancreatic**

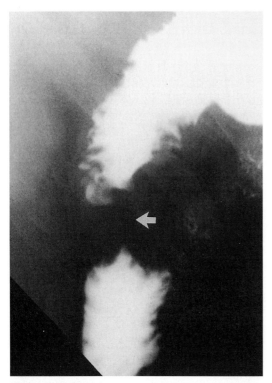

Figure 5–6. Annular pancreas. Single-contrast examination indicates narrowing in the second portion of the duodenum *(arrow)* from encircling pancreatic tissue that has become inflamed.

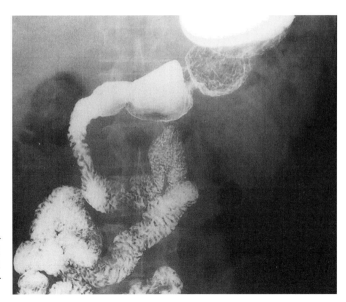

Figure 5–8. Malrotation. Single-contrast examination reveals an abnormal position of the duodenojejunal junction and jejunum, which is abnormally located in the right upper quadrant.

tissue usually are 1 to 2 cm in size with a central dimple that represents a rudimentary duct.

Duodenal diverticula can be either congenital or acquired. They are seen commonly and may be single or multiple and can be located anywhere in the duodenum (Fig. 5–9). Duodenal diverticula are usually of no clinical significance, but they can become inflamed (duodenal diverticulitis), ulcerate, perforate, torque, or contain biliary calculi. Intramural diverticula are thought to represent duodenal webs that have been stretched by peristalsis.

Abnormal **extrinsic deformity** of the duodenum (Fig. 5–10) most commonly occurs from abnormalities of the pancreas, such as annular pancreas, pancreatitis, pancreatic pseudocysts, and pancreatic carcinoma. Abnormalities of the gallbladder and common bile duct as well as lymphadenopathy (usually from lymphoma) can deform the duodenum externally.

Duodenitis

Duodenitis refers to inflammation of the duodenal mucosa. Common causes include

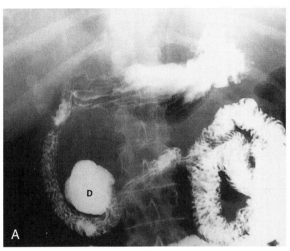

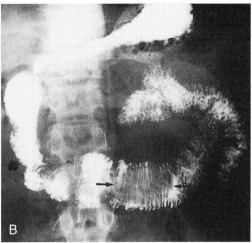

Figure 5–9. Duodenal diverticulosis. Single-contrast upper gastrointestinal series indicates a single large duodenal diverticulum (D) as well as calcified gallstones **(A)** and the "windsock" appearance of an intramural diverticulum *(arrows)* **(B)**.

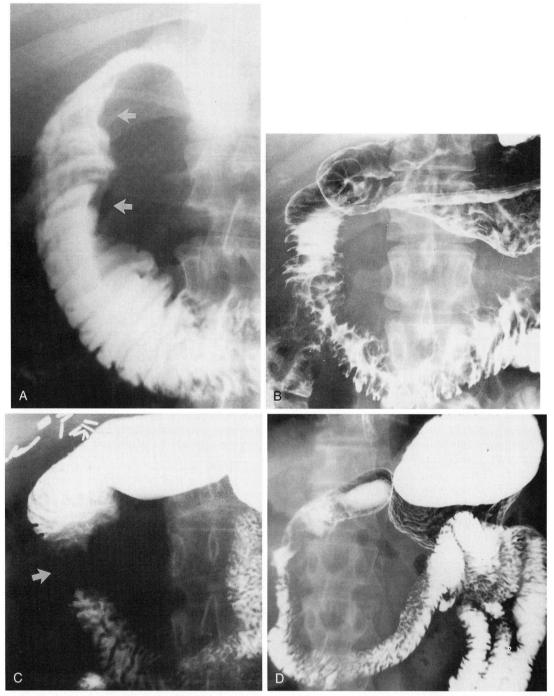

Figure 5–10. Abnormal extrinsic deformities of the duodenum. Single-contrast examinations show various abnormal extrinsic deformities of the duodenum: **A,** Pancreatitis, creating a "reverse 3" impression *(arrows)*. **B,** Pancreatitis with pseudocysts widening the duodenal C-loop. **C,** Pancreatic carcinoma obliterating the duodenal lumen *(arrow)*. **D,** Lymphoma deforming the duodenal C-loop.

Helicobacter pylori infection and nonsteroidal anti-inflammatory drugs. Duodenitis often is found in conjunction with gastritis. Radiographic manifestations of duodenitis include mucosal nodularity, thickening of the duodenal folds, and spasm (Fig. 5–11). As in the stomach, erosions and frank ulcerations may occur. When inflammatory conditions exist, **Brunner gland hyperplasia** may occur. In this condition, the glands of Brun-

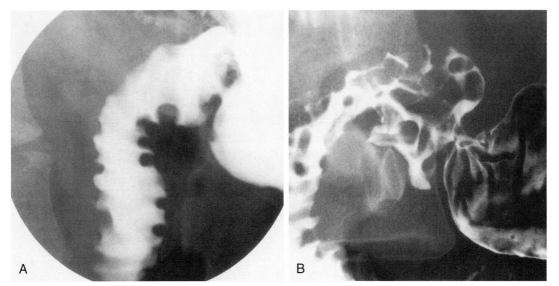

Figure 5–11. Duodenitis. A, Single-contrast examination shows thickening of the duodenal folds. **B,** Mucosal nodularity is seen in another patient with double-contrast examination. These findings are consistent with duodenitis from *H. pylori* infection, Zollinger-Ellison syndrome, or Crohn disease.

ner become hypertrophied and have a nodular appearance.

Involvement of the duodenum with **Crohn disease** is rare. As in other parts of the gastrointestinal system, radiographic findings include aphthous ulcerations, thickening of the mucosal folds, cobblestoning, fibrosis, strictures, and fistula formation (Fig. 5–12).

Peptic Ulcer Disease

As suggested by the term **peptic ulcer disease**, ulcers of the stomach and duodenum often are grouped together as representing the same disease process. Despite the publicity afforded to gastric ulcers, **duodenal ulcers** are more common. Duodenal

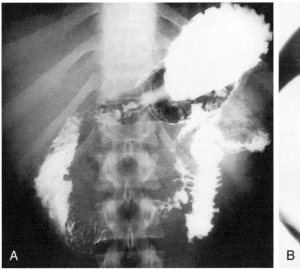

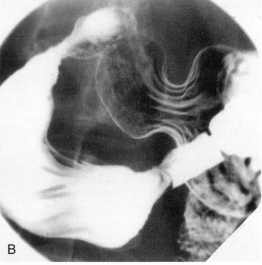

Figure 5–12. Crohn disease. Upper gastrointestinal examinations in two patients reveal findings of Crohn disease. **A,** Thickened and distorted mucosal folds involve the entire duodenum and proximal jejunum in a patient with active disease. **B,** Three strictures in chronic disease: a tapering stricture involving the duodenal bulb and immediate postbulbar segment, a bandlike stricture causing incomplete obstruction at the junction of the third and fourth portions of the duodenum, and a bandlike stricture at the junction of the duodenum and jejunum.

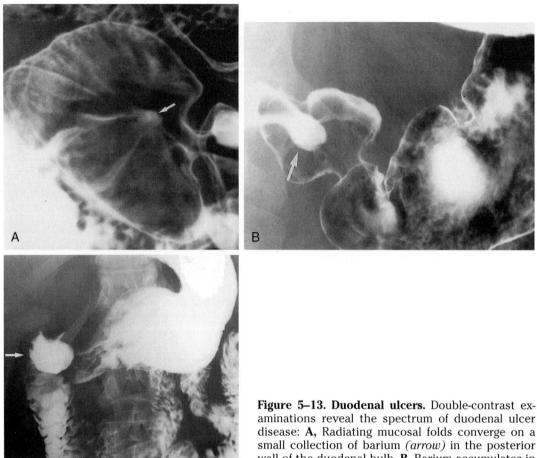

Figure 5–13. Duodenal ulcers. Double-contrast examinations reveal the spectrum of duodenal ulcer disease: **A,** Radiating mucosal folds converge on a small collection of barium *(arrow)* in the posterior wall of the duodenal bulb. **B,** Barium accumulates in a large duodenal ulcer *(arrow)*. **C,** Barium opacifies a giant duodenal ulcer that could be mistaken for the duodenal bulb.

and gastric ulcers share the same causes, with *H. pylori* infection accounting for greater than 90% of duodenal ulcers.

Approximately 95% of duodenal ulcers occur in the bulb. As with gastric ulcers, radiographic features of a duodenal ulcer include persistent collections of barium, radiating mucosal folds, surrounding edema, and abnormal peristalsis (Fig. 5–13). **Giant duodenal ulcers** can replace the bulb and may be mistaken for a deformed bulb. Absence of mucosal folds, aperistalsis, and severe spasm can suggest the diagnosis.

In contrast to gastric ulcers, the location of duodenal ulcers can suggest benignity or malignancy. Most ulcers in the duodenal bulb are benign, whereas postbulbar ulcers should be considered malignant until proved otherwise. Regardless of the initial radiographic appearance, post-treatment follow-up of peptic ulcer disease is recommended to assess for resolution.

Duodenal ulceration may extend through the serosa, perforating into the peritoneum anteriorly or the pancreas posteriorly. Perforation is more common with duodenal ulcers than gastric ulcers. Anterior bulb ulcers perforate into the peritoneum, whereas posterior bulb ulcers can erode into the gastroduodenal artery and cause massive bleeding. Ulcers of the duodenal bulb may resolve with minimal deformity, or an "hourglass" or "cloverleaf" deformity may result (Fig. 5–14). Ulcers in the postbulbar segment often cause severe stricturing.

Benign Neoplasms

Benign neoplasms of the duodenum include lipomas, leiomyomas, adenomatous

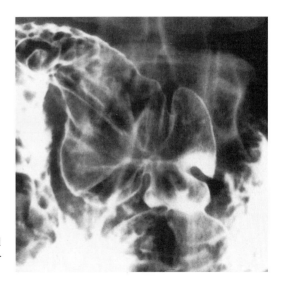

Figure 5–14. "Cloverleaf" deformity. Scarring and spasm of the duodenal bulb can deform the duodenal bulb, giving it a "cloverleaf" appearance.

polyps, villous adenomas, Brunner gland adenomas, and carcinoid tumors. These tumors usually appear as filling defects that often are indistinguishable from each other (Fig. 5–15).

Leiomyomas and **lipomas** occasionally occur as discrete smooth, rounded masses. Leiomyomas have a tendency to ulcerate and can produce anemia and melena.

Adenomatous polyps and **villous adenomas** are seen uncommonly but have a high malignant potential, particularly in the second portion of the duodenum. Villous adenomas tend to be large and bulky and are seen in the periampullary region. **Carcinoid tumors** also are potentially malignant lesions.

Malignant Neoplasms

Primary malignant neoplasms of the duodenum include adenocarcinoma, leiomyosar-

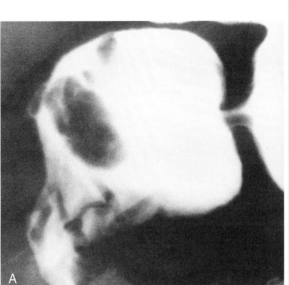

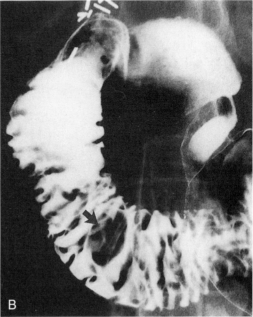

Figure 5–15. Benign duodenal neoplasms. Single-contrast examinations reveal smooth rounded filling defects in the duodenal bulb **(A)** and distal duodenum *(arrow)* **(B).** These lesions subsequently were identified pathologically as an adenomatous polyp and a lymphangioma.

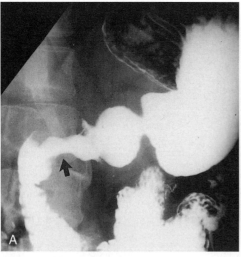 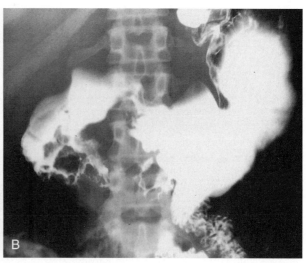

Figure 5–16. Duodenal adenocarcinoma. Single-contrast upper gastrointestinal series displays various appearances of duodenal adenocarcinoma: **A,** Encircling the first portion of the duodenum *(arrow)*; **B,** Deforming the periampullary region.

coma, and lymphoma. **Adenocarcinoma** is the most common malignancy of the duodenum and usually presents as a bulky, ulcerated mass or a circumferential infiltrating mass (Fig. 5–16). Adenocarcinoma of the antrum crosses the pylorus in 5% of cases. **Leiomyosarcoma** of the duodenum is an uncommon tumor that presents as an excavating, ulcerating mass that is large and bulky (Fig. 5–17). **Lymphoma** can appear as a polypoid mass, thickened folds, or ulcerated mass. Lymphoma is known to cross the pylorus from antrum to duodenum in one third of cases.

Metastases to the duodenum may occur from any site by hematogenous seeding. Lymphoma and metastatic carcinoma may involve the peripancreatic and periaortic lymph nodes and enlarge the duodenal sweep and invade directly to a segment of the duodenum (Fig. 5–18). Direct invasion from pancreatic carcinoma to the duodenum is usually in the second portion of the duodenum.

Miscellaneous Conditions

Intramural hematoma of the duodenum characteristically follows blunt trauma to

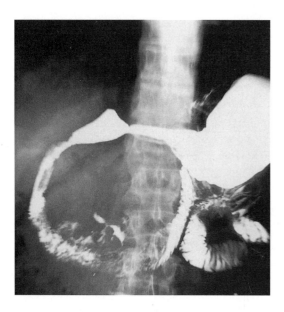

Figure 5–17. Duodenal leiomyosarcoma. Single-contrast upper gastrointestinal series exhibits deformity of the duodenal C-loop and ulceration of the third portion of the duodenum from a leiomyosarcoma.

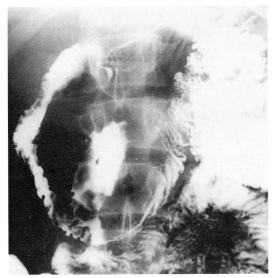

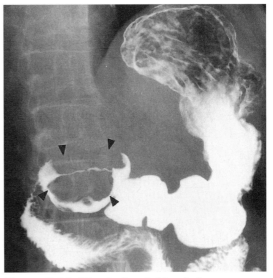

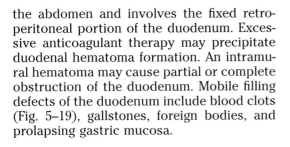

Figure 5–18. Duodenal metastasis. Upper gastro-intestinal series reveals filling of a fistulous tract to the third portion of the duodenum created by metastatic embryonal cell carcinoma.

Figure 5–19. Blood clot. A blood clot creates a large filling defect *(arrows)* in the first portion of the duodenum that expands the lumen.

the abdomen and involves the fixed retro-peritoneal portion of the duodenum. Excessive anticoagulant therapy may precipitate duodenal hematoma formation. An intramural hematoma may cause partial or complete obstruction of the duodenum. Mobile filling defects of the duodenum include blood clots (Fig. 5–19), gallstones, foreign bodies, and prolapsing gastric mucosa.

Suggested Readings

Gore RM, Levine MS, Laufer I: Textbook of Gastrointestinal Radiology, 2nd ed. Philadelphia, WB Saunders, 2000.

Houston JD, Davis M: Fundamentals of Fluoroscopy. Philadelphia, WB Saunders, 2001.

Laufer I, Levine MS, Rubesin SE: Double Contrast Gastrointestinal Radiology, 3rd ed. Philadelphia, WB Saunders, 1999.

Marshak RH, Lindner AE, Maklansky D: Radiology of the Stomach. Philadelphia, WB Saunders, 1983.

SIX

Small Intestine

Michael Davis, M.D., and Jeffrey D. Houston, M.D.

Normal Anatomy

The small intestine includes the duodenum, jejunum, and ileum and averages nearly 3 m in length in vivo. From the ligament of Treitz, the proximal 40% comprises jejunum, and the distal 60% comprises ileum. Most of the jejunum normally is located in the left upper quadrant of the abdomen, whereas the ileum normally occupies much of the pelvis, particularly the right lower quadrant (Fig. 6–1). The terminal ileum communicates with the cecum through the ileocecal valve.

The caliber of the jejunum is slightly larger than the ileum. The transversely oriented **circular folds** (of Kerckring), also known as the **plicae circulares** or **valvulae conniventes,** of the small bowel, are more numerous proximally and progressively disappear by the time the distal ileum is reached. There is no abrupt demarcation between the jejunum and ileum, but rather a gradual transition. The appearance of the valvulae conniventes allows determination of the type of bowel. In the jejunum, the valvulae are prominent and deep, producing a more feathery appearance than the ileum.

Lymphoid follicles contained in the Peyer patches of the distal ileum may be quite prominent in children and young adults. Prominent lymphoid follicles can impart a finely nodular appearance to the terminal ileum (Fig. 6–2).

Imaging Modalities

Indications for radiographic examination of the small intestine include suspected small bowel obstruction, inflammatory bowel disease, malabsorption, gastrointestinal bleeding not diagnosed by previous examination of the upper or lower gastrointestinal tract, benign and malignant neoplasms, unexplained abdominal pain, diarrhea, motility disorders, polyposis syndromes, and small bowel fistulas.

Radiographic examination using an oral contrast agent, usually barium, is a time-proven method for diagnosing a variety of small bowel abnormalities. Examination of the small intestine can be easily botched by improper radiographic technique: too little or too much barium, overly dense barium, and inadequate filming by the radiologist. Meticulous technique is required so that subtle abnormalities may be identified.

Radiologic evaluation of small bowel disease is usually performed by having the patient orally ingest barium or by infusing it through an enteric tube. In rare cases, the small bowel can be evaluated by refluxing contrast retrograde from the colon through the ileocecal valve.

In a conventional **small bowel series**, the patient ingests a specified amount of barium (60% weight volume [w/v]), usually after an upper gastrointestinal series (Fig. 6–3A). Periodic filming of the small intestine is performed as the contrast agent progresses through the bowel loops. The radiologist periodically uses compression technique to separate bowel loops that are overlapped and spot filming to image these bowel segments. When the contrast material has reached the terminal ileum, additional spot filming is done specifically of that area. The examination is concluded when barium reaches the ileocecal valve and cecum.

Enteroclysis (small bowel infusion) is the second routine method used to examine the small intestine (Fig. 6–3B). A nasoenteric tube is placed either at or beyond the duodenojejunal flexure, followed by infusion of barium with a pump or hand injection with syringes. This technique allows for distention of the lumen of the small intestine, permitting a superior anatomic look at the de-

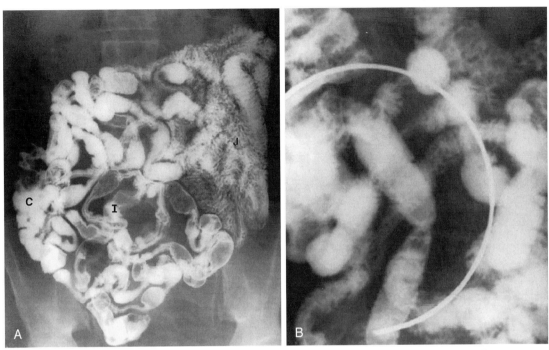

Figure 6–1. Normal anatomy of the small intestine. A, Single-contrast small bowel series demonstrates feathery loops of jejunum (J) in the left upper quadrant and smooth loops of ileum (I) in the right abdomen and pelvis that communicate with the cecum (C). **B,** A normal terminal ileum is visualized with spot compression.

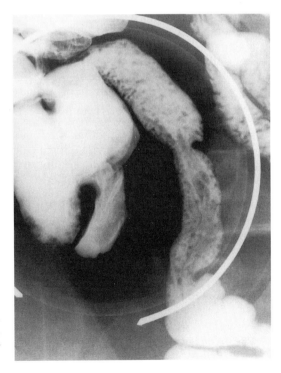

Figure 6–2. Lymphoid follicles. Spot compression view of the terminal ileum reveals multiple small filling defects, representing normal lymphoid follicles in a young adult.

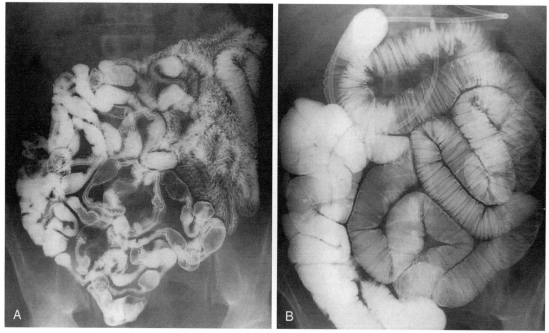

Figure 6–3. Routine small bowel examinations. Normal small bowel series **(A)** and normal double-contrast enteroclysis **(B)**. (From Houston JD, Davis M: Fundamentals of Fluoroscopy. Philadelphia, WB Saunders, 2001.)

tail of the bowel and mucosal folds. This technique can be augmented by following the barium with methylcellulose, a water-like substance that gives a double-contrast effect, allowing visualization through the bowel lumen and the ability to see through other nearby bowel loops.

Computed tomography (CT) of the small intestine has limited applications and is best reserved for further evaluation of already established abnormalities. Imaging can be optimized by completely filling the small bowel with dilute contrast before scanning. CT can be particularly useful in localizing the site of bowel obstruction, suggesting traumatic injury, and identifying enteric duplication cysts. Some institutions are experimenting with CT enteroclysis.

Nuclear medicine imaging of the small bowel is restricted mostly to localization of tumors, Meckel diverticula, or sources of bleeding. In the **Meckel diverticulum scan,** technetium 99m pertechnetate is administered intravenously, and sequential images are obtained to localize the diverticulum on the basis of uptake of the radionuclide within the ectopic gastric mucosa. **Gastrointestinal bleeding studies** are performed most commonly with technetium 99m–labeled red blood cells. The **Schilling test**

can be used for evaluating patients with pernicious anemia or malabsorption by examining small bowel absorption of vitamin B_{12} by administering cobalt 57–labeled vitamin B_{12} and measuring a 24-hour urine sample for excreted activity.

Ultrasonography can be used in the evaluation of intussusception, particularly in children. Duplication cysts are examined initially with ultrasound because they often present as palpable masses.

Structural Abnormalities

Congenital abnormalities of the small intestine include atresia, stenosis, duplication anomalies, malrotation, and Meckel diverticula.

Atresia is twice as common in the jejunum and ileum as in the duodenum. There is nearly equal distribution between the jejunum and ileum, and jejunoileal atresia can be associated with other anomalies, such as malrotation and volvulus. In cases of proximal atresia, sufficient succus entericus is produced by the distal bowel to result in a normal-diameter colon, whereas a distal atresia commonly produces a microcolon.

Jejunoileal stenosis is much less common than atresia.

Duplications of the small bowel are rare and result from abnormal recanalization. Most duplications are cystic, but tubular duplications also can occur. Duplications are prone to develop on the mesenteric side of the bowel. **Enteric duplication cysts** are less likely to communicate with the lumen than the tubular variety and can cause obstruction. The tubular varieties are more likely to contain ectopic gastric mucosa.

As previously discussed, **malrotation** occurs from aberrant extracoelomic rotation of the bowel during fetal development and can cause midgut volvulus, most commonly in pediatric patients. Incidentally diagnosed rotational anomalies of the small intestine are usually of no clinical significance in adults (Fig. 6–4).

Meckel diverticula occur in about 2% of the population. They are congenital in origin and occur within 1 m of the ileocecal valve (Fig. 6–5). Most diverticula measure 1 to 5 cm in length. The radiologic diagnosis of Meckel diverticulum is difficult, with enteroclysis being the barium method of choice. Complications include hematochezia, melena, diverticulum inversion with intussusception and obstruction, and small bowel

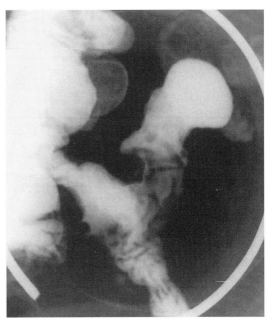

Figure 6–5. Meckel diverticulum. Single-contrast examination allows filling of a Meckel diverticulum arising superomedially from the terminal ileum.

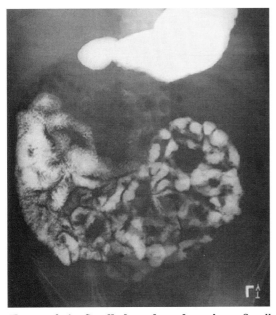

Figure 6–4. Small bowel malrotation. Small bowel series shows malrotation of the small intestine, with the jejunum abnormally located in the right upper quadrant of the abdomen.

obstruction from twisting of bowel loops around the vitelline duct remnant. Scintigraphic studies can detect ectopic gastric mucosa and bleeding from the diverticulum. Bleeding occurs from peptic ulceration of the unprotected mucosa in the diverticulum and particularly from ulceration within the ectopic gastric mucosa. Most bleeding episodes occur in patients under 10 years of age and rarely after 30 years of age. Concretions can form in Meckel diverticula and cause impaction, followed by diverticulitis, gangrene, and perforation.

Diverticula of the small intestine are acquired and usually single or few in number, but extensive diverticulosis of the small intestine occasionally is encountered (Fig. 6–6). Most small bowel diverticula are located in the jejunum. Complications from diverticula include bleeding, obstruction, diverticulitis (with perforation and abscess formation), and malabsorption.

Small bowel obstruction is caused by mechanical blockage of the intestinal lumen that can occur from a myriad of conditions, including adhesions, hernias, neoplasms, intussusception, volvulus, foreign bodies, and inflammatory processes. Small bowel obstruction often appears radiographically as intestinal distention, which is defined as be-

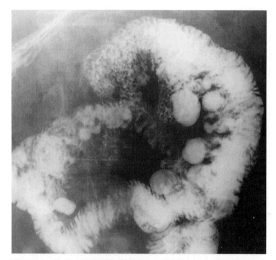

Figure 6–6. Jejunal diverticulosis. Single-contrast examination illustrates diverticula of varying sizes distributed throughout the jejunum.

ing greater than 3 cm in diameter (Fig. 6–7). Differential air-fluid levels can produce a "stepladder" or "inverted U" pattern on upright radiographs. The "string-of-pearls" sign refers to a row of small bubbles of gas that are trapped between the valvulae conni-

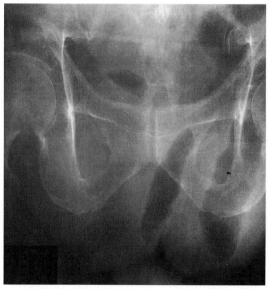

Figure 6–8. Inguinal hernia. Conventional radiograph of the abdomen shows prolapse of a gas-filled loop of small bowel through the left inguinal canal into the scrotum.

ventes, with the remainder of the bowel loop filled with fluid.

Small bowel hernias can be internal or external. Most small bowel hernias are external and consist of inguinal, femoral, obturator, and abdominal wall hernias (Fig. 6–8). Abdominal wall hernias include umbilical,

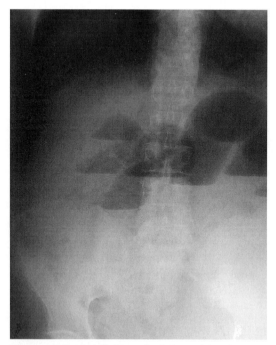

Figure 6–7. Small bowel obstruction. Conventional radiograph of the abdomen shows dilation of multiple loops of small bowel, with differential air-fluid levels, resulting from obstruction.

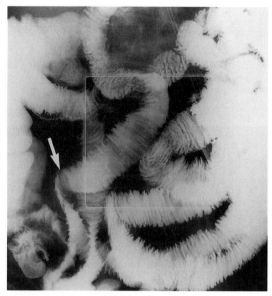

Figure 6–9. Adhesions. Single-contrast enteroclysis reveals a linear adhesion *(arrow)* partially obstructing the jejunum.

incisional, and spigelian hernias. The **spigelian hernia** is located between the external and internal oblique muscles and is caused by weakness of the abdominal muscle sheaths.

Adhesions account for about half of mechanical obstructions (Fig. 6–9), with most adhesions arising from prior abdominal surgery. **Gallstone ileus** is an uncommon entity in which the small bowel (usually the ileum) becomes obstructed by a gallstone that passes through the biliary system or erodes into the alimentary canal (Fig. 6–10).

A variety of conditions can produce an **adynamic ileus,** which can mimic obstruction clinically and radiologically, by interfering with normal peristalsis (Fig. 6–11). Causes of adynamic ileus include the postoperative state, ischemia, inflammatory processes, drugs, neuromuscular disorders, collagen vascular diseases, and diabetes.

Inflammatory Bowel Disease

Crohn disease (regional enteritis) is a chronic inflammatory condition of the gastrointestinal tract that may have genetic and

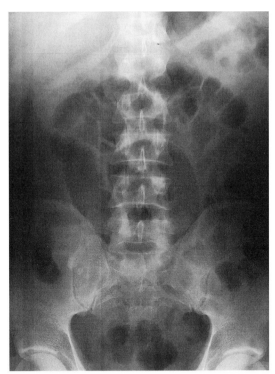

Figure 6–11. Adynamic ileus. Conventional radiograph of the abdomen exhibits gaseous distention of several loops of small bowel. Small bowel obstruction can have a similar appearance.

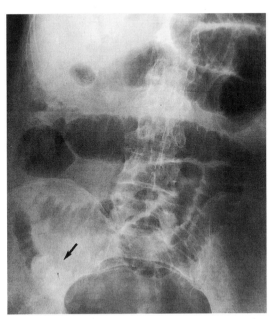

Figure 6–10. Gallstone ileus. Conventional radiograph of the abdomen indicates abnormal dilation of several loops of obstructed small bowel. The bowel gas abruptly terminates in the right lower quadrant at the site of impaction of a calcified gallstone *(arrow).*

environmental links. Cigarette smoking, dietary factors, viral infection, and mycobacterial infection are some of the many suspected causative factors. The peak incidence of onset is between 15 and 25 years of age. Crohn disease also can strike in later years, usually between ages 55 and 60.

The small bowel is involved in 80% of patients (35% ileitis, 45% ileocolitis) with the terminal ileum the most common site. Isolated colitis occurs in 20% of patients, most often in the right colon, although pancolitis sometimes can occur. The usual symptoms are abdominal pain, fever, nausea, vomiting, diarrhea (sometimes bloody), and weight loss.

The radiographic appearance of Crohn disease of the small bowel is varied (Fig. 6–12) and can be divided into two phases: the prestenotic phase and the stenotic phase. The **prestenotic phase** (nonstenotic phase) findings include blunting, flattening, distortion, straightening, and thickening of the mucosal folds as a result of obstructive lymphedema. These changes are followed by the formation of **aphthous erosions** (aph-

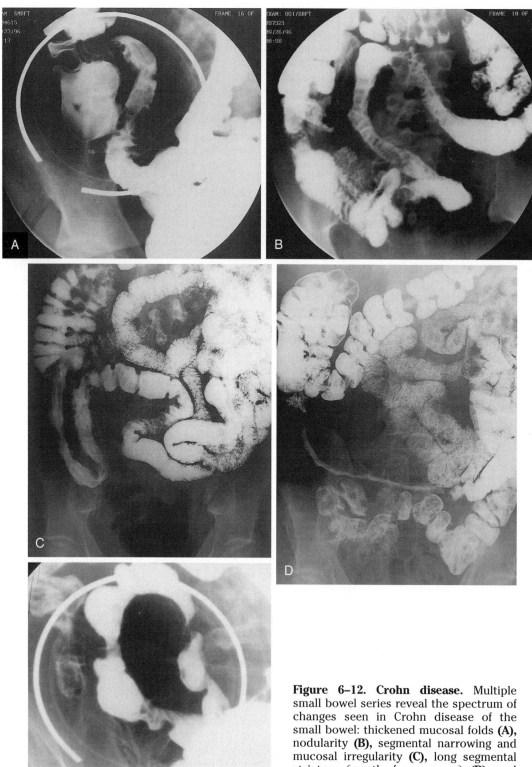

Figure 6–12. Crohn disease. Multiple small bowel series reveal the spectrum of changes seen in Crohn disease of the small bowel: thickened mucosal folds **(A),** nodularity **(B),** segmental narrowing and mucosal irregularity **(C),** long segmental stricture (mostly from spasm) **(D),** and multifocal strictures of the terminal ileum with intervening areas of dilation between the strictures **(E).**

thae), which can coalesce to form linear ulcers. Some of these ulcers may penetrate deeply into the wall, producing stellate or "rose thorn" shapes that are seen best in profile. Serpiginous ulcers separated by areas of edema create the appearance of **cobblestoning.** Hyperplastic mucosal islands surrounded by denuded mucosa are termed **inflammatory pseudopolyps.**

When healing occurs and new mucosa is formed, the inflammatory pseudopolyps become **postinflammatory polyps.** A hallmark of Crohn disease is the presence of **skip lesions,** which are diseased segments interposed between normal segments of bowel. When the mesenteric side of the bowel wall is affected severely, often extending into the mesentery and followed by scarring, the antimesenteric side may bulge outward to form sacculations or **pseudodiverticula.**

With continued bowel wall thickening and further mesenteric involvement, extra mesenteric fat forms, and the affected bowel loops become separated and the normal loops displaced. Mesenteric lymphadenopathy is present at this stage.

In the **stenotic phase,** the bowel lumen is narrowed over varying distances. The terminal ileum may be so narrowed from spasm that it is referred to as a **string sign,** so named because it appears to resemble a frayed cotton string. The normal bowel loops proximal to the strictures may become dilated. Strictures are seen in about 20% of patients with Crohn disease affecting the small bowel. Because of the high rate of recurrence of the disease (75% in 1 year) after surgical resection for obstruction, it now is recommended that strictureplasty be done.

Complications other than small bowel obstruction include fistulas, intramural sinus tracts, abscesses, perforation (uncommon), hydronephrosis, and toxic megacolon (when the colon is involved). Adenocarcinoma is a grave sequela of Crohn disease. The actual incidence of cancer is uncertain, but it is known that younger patients with longstanding disease in the terminal ileum are at highest risk. Preoperative radiologic detection is rare owing to the absence of the usual findings of small bowel carcinoma. Extraintestinal manifestations of Crohn disease involve many systems. There is an increase in gallstones (from malabsorption of bile salts in the terminal ileum), fatty liver, sclerosing cholangitis, and cholangiocarcinoma.

Infectious Enteritis

Caused by food-borne infection with the gram-negative rod *Yersinia enterocolitica,* **yersiniosis** presents with abdominal pain, mostly in the right lower quadrant, and mimics appendicitis. The radiographic findings are limited to the distal ileum with thickened mucosal folds, nodularity, and aphthae. This infection mimics Crohn disease with the exception that fistulas are not formed, and there is no permanent stenosis.

The ileocecal area is the most common site for intestinal **tuberculosis.** The radiographic findings are not specific but include mucosal nodularity with eventual effacement of the folds, ulcerations, luminal narrowing, and possible fistula formation. The cecum almost always is involved and, with time, a "coned" cecum may become evident (Fig. 6–13).

Salmonellosis comprises infection by any

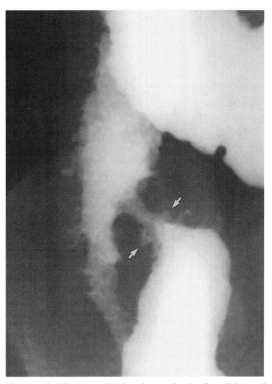

Figure 6–13. Intestinal tuberculosis. Small bowel series shows narrowing of the terminal ileum, with several ulcerations *(arrows).* A "coned" cecum with multiple small ulcerations is apparent. A fibrotic terminal ileum that communicates through a patent ileocecal valve with a contracted cecum and ascending colon is known as the *Stierlin sign.*

of a large group of gram-negative bacilli of the *Salmonella* species. Clinical presentation generally involves diarrhea, fever, and myalgias. Radiographic findings usually include shallow ulcerations of the terminal ileum and proximal ascending colon.

Campylobacter enteritis, caused by the microaerophilic gram-negative rod *Campylobacter jejuni*, is a common cause of waterborne bacterial diarrhea. Radiographic findings are usually confined to the distal ileum and the proximal ascending colon, where distortion of the mucosal folds occurs with nodularity and spiculation.

First recognized in 1907, **Whipple disease** was a mysterious condition. The causative organism was not cultured until 1999. Bacteria, long known to exist in intestinal biopsy specimens, have been identified by genetic analysis (polymerase chain reaction) as *Tropheryma whippelii*, a gram-positive actinomycete. Most of the patients are middle-aged men with symptoms of malabsorption, fever, weight loss, chronic uveitis, endocarditis, arthralgia, lymphadenopathy, and skin pigmentation. Hypersecretion often occurs and creates hypoalbuminemia. The radiographic findings are mainly distortion and thickening of the mucosal folds of the duodenum and jejunum.

Histoplasmosis, caused by the fungus *Histoplasma capsulatum*, usually involves the lungs and skin, but also may affect the gastrointestinal tract. This disease usually occurs with debilitating illnesses and characteristically involves the ileocecal region. Radiographic findings consist of mucosal granularity, irregular thickened folds, luminal narrowing, stricture, and occasional fistula formation.

The water-borne protozoan *Giardia lamblia* causes **giardiasis,** an infection that produces diarrhea and abdominal pain. Radiographic findings include mucosal thickening and nodularity, with increased secretions in the duodenum and jejunum. The bowel lumen may be widened, and hypermotility may be present (Fig. 6–14).

Strongyloidiasis, caused by the nematode *Strongyloides stercoralis*, is mostly a disease of the tropics. The larvae enter through the skin and migrate through the venous system to the lungs, where they penetrate alveoli, then migrate to the small bowel. Radiographic findings are motility disturbances, effacement of the mucosal folds with luminal narrowing, and occasional dilation.

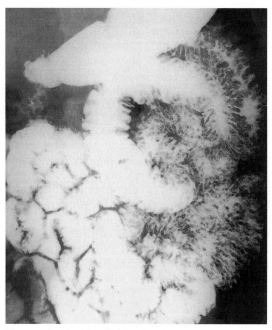

Figure 6–14. Giardiasis. Small bowel series illustrates diffusely thickened jejunal folds in the left upper quadrant and left midabdomen. Signs of hypermotility and hypersecretion often are present.

Ascaris lumbricoides is a nematode found in the intestine in a significant portion of the world's population. Originating from ingested eggs, the larvae emerge in the duodenum, penetrate the mucosa, enter the portal venous system, and continue through the liver to the lungs. The larvae then migrate to the pharynx and are swallowed, maturing in the small intestine. Radiographic findings of **ascariasis** include long, linear filling defects within the intestine (Fig. 6–15). The worms may be 20 to 30 cm in length. Occasionally the worms' intestinal tract may be filled with barium.

Cytomegalovirus enteritis almost always is confined to patients with immunodeficiency or immunosuppressive disorders. This infection may involve any segment of the gastrointestinal tract, with the small bowel being involved infrequently. In the ileum, cytomegalovirus infection may be manifested initially as lymphoid hyperplasia, followed by edematous thickening of the mucosa and small discrete ulcerations. In the more advanced stage, deeper ulcerations, mucosal effacement, and bowel wall thickening may be seen (Fig. 6–16). In some patients, the infected bowel has **aneurysmal dilation** similar to that seen in lymphoma.

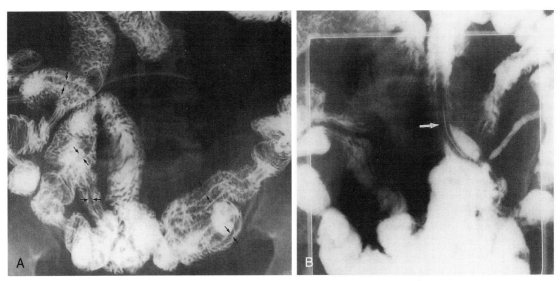

Figure 6–15. Ascariasis. Small bowel series in two patients reveal multiple serpiginous filling defects in the jejunum *(arrows)* **(A)** as well as ingested contrast within the intestine of the worm *(arrow)* **(B).**

Diffuse Intestinal Disease

Hypoproteinemia of any cause results in edematous changes throughout long segments of intestine. Edema produces thickening and straightening of the mucosal folds (Fig. 6–17). The excessive secretions of the stomach in **Ménètrier disease** cause hypoproteinemia, with thickened and straight-

ened folds in the jejunum. There is no known primary involvement of the small bowel.

The changes of **intestinal lymphangiectasia** are from loss of protein owing to lymphatic obstruction. Radiographically, there is generalized thickening and straightening of the small bowel folds.

Mastocytosis is a rare disease that is characterized by cutaneous accumulation of

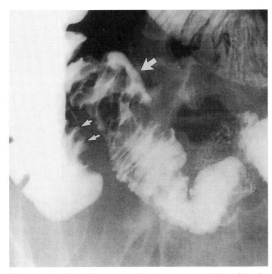

Figure 6–16. Cytomegalovirus enteritis. Single-contrast examination in a patient with acquired immunodeficiency syndrome shows thickened folds in the terminal ileum, a large deep ulceration *(large arrow)*, and involvement of the medial wall of the cecum *(small arrows)*.

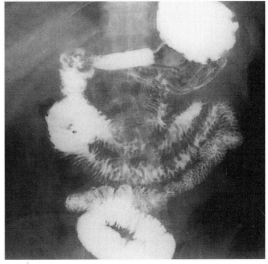

Figure 6–17. Hypoproteinemia. Single-contrast upper gastrointestinal series displays changes of submucosal edema of long segments of small intestine, with thickening and straightening of the mucosal folds.

mast cells. Approximately 10% of patients develop the systemic form, in which mast cells infiltrate other organs, including the gastrointestinal tract. Hepatosplenomegaly is common, and 70% of patients develop bone lesions. Gastrointestinal mastocytosis may present clinically as malabsorption. Radiographically, there is distortion and thickening of the mucosal folds, particularly in the jejunum. A tiny nodular pattern sometimes is seen.

Changes of **radiation enteritis** are seen mostly in women treated for gynecologic malignancies. Symptoms of radiation injury often manifest 6 to 24 months after radiation therapy and are due to ischemia from damage to the gut arterioles. Radiographic findings include thickening and straightening of the mucosal folds, stricture, kinking and angulation with matting of the small intestinal loops, obstruction, and fistula formation (Fig. 6–18).

Progressive systemic sclerosis (scleroderma) often involves the small intestine and results from collagen deposition and fibrosis. Radiographically, there is hypomotility, and the intestinal tract becomes mark-

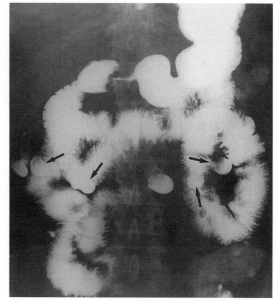

Figure 6–19. Progressive systemic sclerosis (scleroderma). Small bowel series reveals dilation of the intestinal lumen with a "stack of coins" appearance. The folds themselves are of normal thickness. Multiple pseudodiverticula are present *(arrows)*.

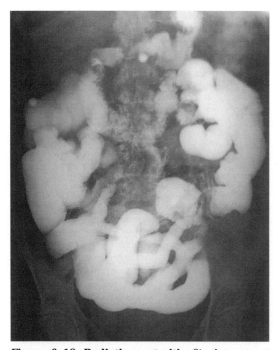

Figure 6–18. Radiation enteritis. Single-contrast examination illustrates narrowing of the bowel lumen and obliteration of the mucosal folds, with matting of the loops in a patient with chronic radiation enteritis.

edly dilated with thin stretched mucosal folds that give the small bowel a "stack of coins" appearance. Eccentric sacculations that represent wide-mouthed **pseudodiverticula** are suggestive of the disease (Fig. 6–19).

Celiac disease (gluten-sensitive enteropathy or nontropical sprue) is an immune-mediated chronic disease in which the small bowel mucosa is damaged by gluten, a proteinaceous grain constituent containing a water-insoluble protein called *gliadin* that appears to be the offending agent. This disease has a genetic predisposition (HLA B8) and is most common in individuals of European origin. This malabsorption syndrome exhibits intestinal dilation, loss of mucosal folds in the jejunum, and an increased number of mucosal folds in the ileum (*jejunization*) (Fig. 6–20). Increased fluid content may cause precipitation of barium. Intussusception (discussed later) is known to occur in celiac disease, and intestinal lymphoma and carcinoma are known complications. **Tropical sprue** is a celiac-like disease that occurs almost exclusively in the tropics, in which bacterial overgrowth and toxin release has been implicated as the cause.

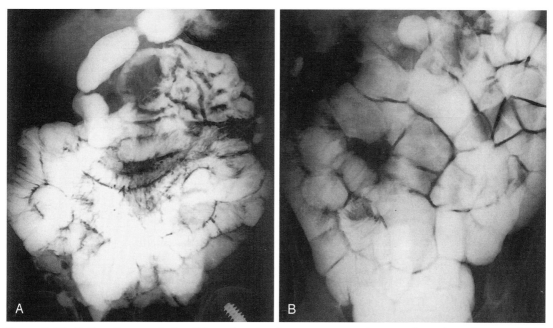

Figure 6–20. Celiac disease. A, Small bowel series demonstrates an increased number of mucosal folds (jejunization) in the ileum. **B,** Single-contrast enteroclysis shows decreased number of the mucosal folds and dilation.

In addition to the stomach, the small bowel is involved significantly by **Zollinger-Ellison syndrome**. This syndrome develops from excessive gastrin secretion, usually from a pancreatic gastrinoma. Gastrin induces hypersecretion of acidic gastric fluid, with enlargement of the folds in the stomach, duodenum, and jejunum. The initial onset may be one to multiple ulcers of the stomach, duodenum, and jejunum. The mucosal folds usually are thick and straight, and the lumen is wide from the voluminous secretions.

Graft-versus-host disease can be a fatal complication of bone marrow transplantation. Allogeneic graft leukocytes can attack the cells of the small intestine. In severe cases, total sloughing of the mucosa can occur. Malabsorption owing to chronic injury may ensue. Radiographically, there is hypermotility, thickening and effacement of mucosal folds, mural thickening with resulting luminal narrowing, and excessive intraluminal fluid (Fig. 6–21).

Ischemic enteritis occurs when there is insufficient blood flow to the small bowel. Acute infarction may be produced by arterial or venous occlusion, and damage occurs within minutes of cessation of perfusion. Within an hour, superficial epithelium is denuded, with progressive involvement of deeper layers. If timely reperfusion occurs, mucosal damage may be reversed after 1 week of healing. Chronic ischemia usually is due to atherosclerosis and is encountered

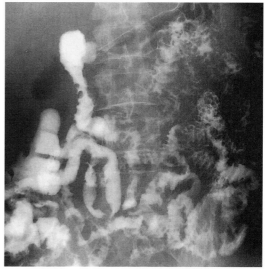

Figure 6–21. Graft-versus-host disease. Single-contrast examination reveals narrowing of the intestinal lumen, wall thickening, and effacement of the mucosal folds. These findings are seen most commonly in the mid to distal ileum.

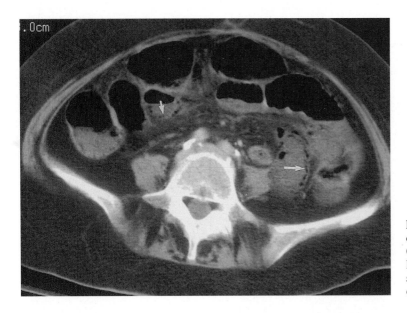

Figure 6–22. Small bowel ischemia. Axial noncontrasted CT of the pelvis illustrates dilation of multiple loops of small bowel with scattered areas of intramural air *(arrows).*

less commonly. Mural thickening from edema and hemorrhage can be seen radiographically (Fig. 6–22). **Shock bowel** is often seen as a result of global hypoperfusion in the setting of trauma. The small bowel becomes diffusely dilated, and the wall becomes thickened (Fig. 6–23).

Benign Neoplasms

Small bowel tumors account for less than 5% of gastrointestinal neoplasms, with benign and malignant tumors being divided equally. Benign tumors are found equally in men and women, usually between 50 and 80 years of age. Symptoms of benign small bowel tumors are bowel obstruction and bleeding.

Adenomas may be seen anywhere in the small intestine, but more often occur proximally in the duodenum and jejunum. They are usually single, but multiple adenomas occasionally occur outside of the polyposis syndromes. Adenomas are initially small, smooth, and sessile, but with growth can ulcerate and cause bleeding. They are premalignant, especially in the duodenum, particularly in the periampullary region.

Other benign tumors of the small intestine

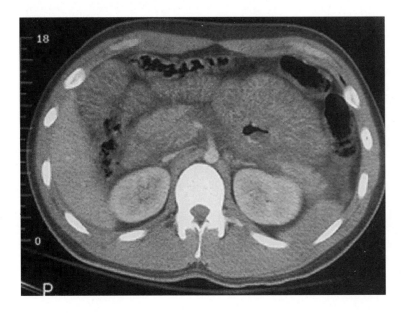

Figure 6–23. Shock bowel. Axial CT with bowel contrast displays marked bowel wall thickening as well as diminished caliber of the aorta and a slitlike appearance of the inferior vena cava, resulting from hypoperfusion.

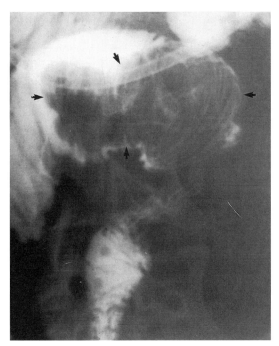

Figure 6–24. Leiomyoma. Small bowel series demonstrates a large filling defect *(arrow)*, representing a leiomyoma, behind which is a large bulky mass with the coiled spring–like appearance of mucosal folds that represent an intussusception.

are of mesenchymal origin and include leiomyoma, lipoma, fibroma, neurofibroma, hemangioma, and lymphangioma. Most of these lesions occur singly, but they may be multiple. The **leiomyoma** is the most common benign small bowel tumor and can develop toward the bowel lumen (endoenteric) or away from the lumen (exoenteric) (Fig. 6–24). The **lipoma** is the second most common benign small bowel tumor and is found more often in the ileum. Lipomas are usually intramural, smooth, and sessile, but they can become pedunculated and cause intussusception. The lesions may ulcerate and bleed. Lipomas, hemangiomas, and lymphangiomas tend to be compressible.

Peutz-Jeghers syndrome is an autosomal dominant disease that features multiple hamartomatous polyps in the stomach, small bowel, and colon. More hamartomas occur in the jejunum than in the ileum. As with other small bowel tumors, these lesions may ulcerate, bleed, and, if pedunculated, cause intussusception.

Another hamartomatous syndrome is **Cowden disease** (multiple hamartoma syn-drome). Patients with Cowden disease have multiple system abnormalities, including mucocutaneous lesions and thyroid, breast, and genitourinary abnormalities in addition to tumors of the gastrointestinal tract. These small bowel tumors are considered hamartomas. They can occur throughout the gastrointestinal tract but are least common in the small intestine. Most of these polyps are less than 5 mm in diameter, and this size requires meticulous technique for identification.

In the **familial polyposis syndrome,** adenomatous polyps occur in the stomach, small intestine, and colon. Discovery usually occurs after adolescence when the tumors grow and bleed. The potential for development of adenocarcinoma in the colon is 100%, ultimately requiring colectomy. Screening for polyps in family members is mandatory. Adenomas of the stomach have a premalignant potential, but the tumors in the periampullary region have a high malignant potential. In this syndrome, adenomas of the jejunum and the ileum usually are small and multiple and have a lower malignant potential than duodenal adenomas.

Cronkhite-Canada syndrome is an uncommon polyposis syndrome of hamartomas occurring in the stomach, small intestine, and colon. This disease is unique among the polyposis syndromes because it is not inherited. Patients with this disease have ectodermal findings that ultimately lead to discovery of intestinal polyps.

Malignant Neoplasms

The most common malignant tumor of the small bowel is actually a secondary tumor, metastasis. The frequency of primary small intestinal malignancies in decreasing order is: malignant carcinoid (41%), adenocarcinoma (24%), lymphoma (22%), sarcoma (11%), and other (2%).

Carcinoid tumors arise from enterochromaffin cells, with most arising in the gastrointestinal tract. Carcinoid is found in the appendix (50%) and in the distal ileum (35%), and the remainder are scattered throughout the gastrointestinal tract. Carcinoid tumors are multiple in half of all cases. Most small bowel carcinoids are asymptomatic, but when present the most common symptom is episodic abdominal pain. Because these tumors rarely ulcerate, bleeding is uncommon, but it can occur if ischemia from mesenteric involvement is severe.

By the time of discovery, up to 80% of ileal carcinoids have metastasized to local lymph nodes, mesentery, or liver. Carcinoid tumors are difficult to diagnose radiographically when they are less than 2 cm in diameter. Initially, they appear as smooth, round mural masses that protrude toward the bowel lumen (Fig. 6–25). At this stage, they have no distinguishing characteristics and resemble other mesenchymal tumors. With growth, the tumor spreads to the serosa and mesentery and protrudes more into the bowel lumen.

As hormones are released, a desmoplastic process in the mesentery ensues that obstructs vessels and causes edema, ischemia, stricture, twisting, and separation of bowel loops with obstruction and bleeding. Mesenteric metastases appear on CT as a central mesenteric mass from which dense strands radiate outward toward the bowel loops, often creating a spoke-wheel appearance. The central mass sometimes calcifies. The **carcinoid syndrome** usually does not occur without hepatic metastases, in which hormones are released into the hepatic veins and thus into the systemic circulation. High levels of serotonin and other metabolic products can cause right-sided endocardial fibrosis, leading to pulmonary valve stenosis and tricuspid valve regurgitation.

Primary adenocarcinomas of the small intestine are relatively rare compared with their incidence in the stomach and colon.

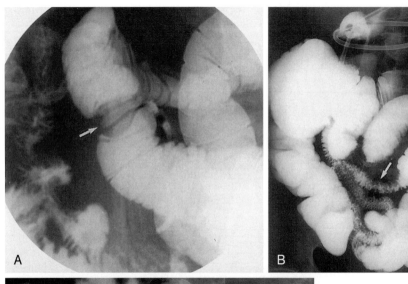

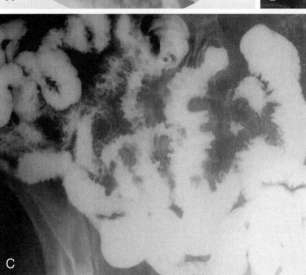

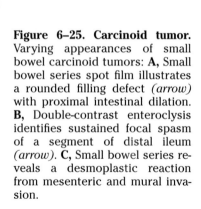

Figure 6–25. Carcinoid tumor. Varying appearances of small bowel carcinoid tumors: **A,** Small bowel series spot film illustrates a rounded filling defect *(arrow)* with proximal intestinal dilation. **B,** Double-contrast enteroclysis identifies sustained focal spasm of a segment of distal ileum *(arrow)*. **C,** Small bowel series reveals a desmoplastic reaction from mesenteric and mural invasion.

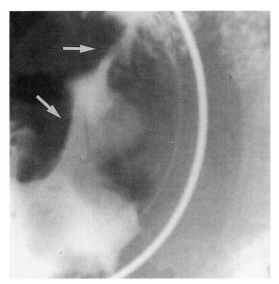

Figure 6–26. Adenocarcinoma. Spot compression view from a small bowel series exhibits a large necrotic mass *(arrows)* in the fourth portion of the duodenum.

They are found more commonly in the jejunum than in the ileum. Their appearance matches adenocarcinomas found elsewhere in the bowel and can be polypoid, ulcerating, or infiltrating (Fig. 6–26).

Non-Hodgkin lymphoma of the small bowel is uncommon in the general population, but it is seen in increasing numbers in patients with human immunodeficiency virus, acquired immunodeficiency syndrome, and celiac disease. Radiographically, non-Hodgkin lymphoma has different presentations: multiple small nodules, a polypoid mass that mimics adenocarcinoma, infiltration of long segments of bowel wall with narrowing of the lumen, and occasionally aneurysmal dilation of the lumen owing to outward proliferation and destruction of nerve plexuses (Fig. 6–27). Non-Hodgkin lymphoma may ulcerate and form fistulas. The variable appearance requires differentiation from adenocarcinoma, metastatic disease, and Crohn disease.

Kaposi sarcoma is an angiogenic neoplasm composed of endothelial and spindle cells. The infective agent is human herpesvirus 8 (HHV-8), and the incidence of HHV-8 infection is highest in populations at risk for Kaposi sarcoma: male homosexuals and transplant recipients. Visceral dissemination is present in more than 50% of patients with skin lesions. The lesions can occur from the oropharynx to the rectum and are usually 1 to 2 cm in diameter, are smooth or nodular, and may show umbilication defects. When present in the small bowel, intussusception may develop. Adenopathy can be seen in the mesentery, retroperitoneum, and pelvis. On contrasted CT, the lymph nodes enhance because of the high degree of vascularity.

Leiomyosarcomas account for a small portion of primary malignancies found in the small intestine. It is a tumor of smooth muscle origin that includes the bowel wall and arteries. Only a few leiomyosarcomas develop from a leiomyoma; the remainder develop from smooth muscle, but the instigating event is unknown. These tumors usually grow to a large size before discovery, when there is mass effect on other organs, intussusception, or bleeding from tumor necrosis (Fig. 6–28). The tumor is often largely exophytic and occasionally does not communicate with the bowel lumen. When a necrotic mass greater than 5 cm in diameter is encountered, leiomyosarcoma should be considered. CT may be able to differentiate leiomyosarcoma from leiomyoma, with the former often greater than 5 cm in size and having a lobulated contour, heterogeneous enhancement, mesenteric fat infiltration, ulceration, regional lymphadenopathy, and exophytic location.

Metastases are the most common small bowel malignancies, accounting for more than half of all small bowel tumors. The most common metastatic lesions are breast carcinoma, lung carcinoma, and melanoma. Other tumors include gastric, renal, pancreatic, ovarian, and uterine malignancies. These lesions can be spread by hematogenous, lymphatic, or contiguous spread. The radiographic appearances of metastases are varied (Fig. 6–29). Hematogenous metastasis becomes radiographically manifest as an ulcerated mass. Melanoma may be seen as multiple "target lesions" throughout the small intestine. Contiguous spread and intra-abdominal seeding of tumor becomes radiographically apparent by mass effect as well as tethering and serrated margins of the bowel wall.

Miscellaneous Conditions

Intussusception refers to the prolapse of one part of the bowel (intussusceptum) into

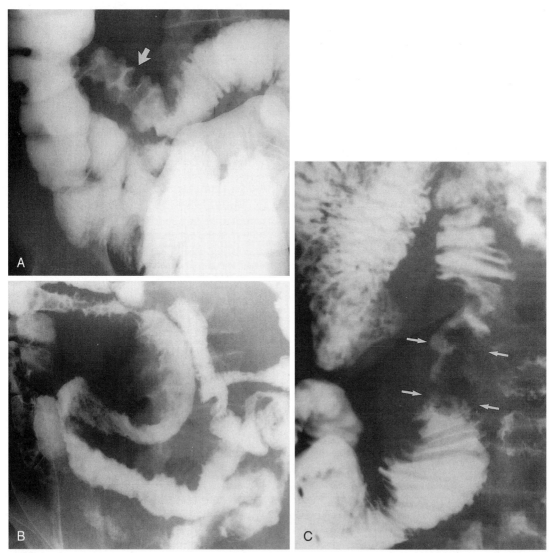

Figure 6–27. Non-Hodgkin lymphoma. Varying appearances of small bowel lymphoma include: **A,** Thickened and nodular mucosal folds in the terminal ileum *(arrow)*. **B,** Marked distortion of mucosa occurring over long segments of the terminal ileum. **C,** Annular constriction of the bowel lumen *(arrows)*.

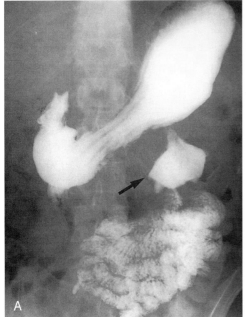

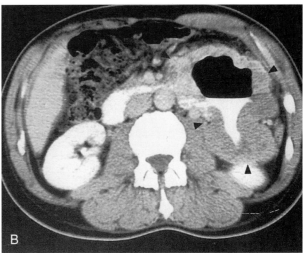

Figure 6–28. Leiomyosarcoma. A, Upper gastrointestinal series shows a large area of necrosis involving the proximal jejunum *(arrow)*. **B,** Axial contrasted CT shows severe circumferential thickening of the wall and an air-fluid level in a patient with a necrotic primary leiomyosarcoma.

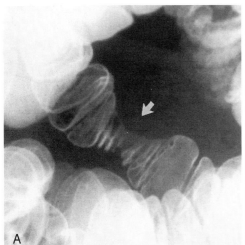

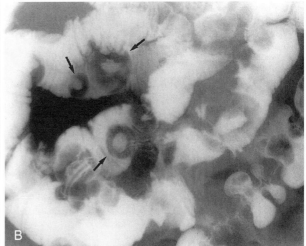

Figure 6–29. Metastatic disease. Varying appearances of small bowel metastases include: **A,** Focal luminal narrowing *(arrow)* from serosal attachment of metastatic nodules from pancreatic carcinoma. **B,** Multiple "target" lesions *(arrows)* from melanoma. **C,** Fine serrations of the wall *(arrows)* from serosal involvement.

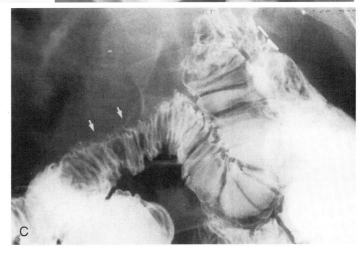

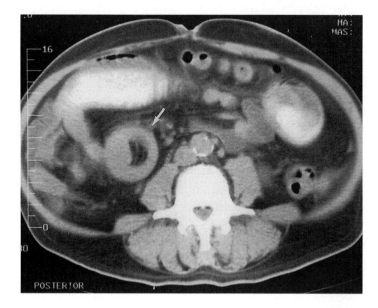

Figure 6–30. Intussusception. Axial CT of the abdomen reveals the "pseudo-kidney" sign *(arrow)* in a case of ileoileal intussusception, with an area of central low attenuation representing invaginated mesenteric fat, and proximally dilated contrast-filled bowel.

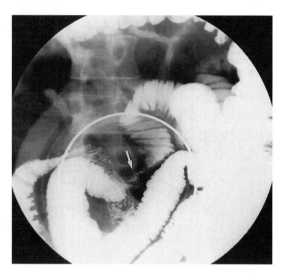

Figure 6–31. Trauma. Spot compression view of a single-contrast enteroclysis reveals a focal area of marked luminal narrowing resulting from a mural hematoma *(arrow)*.

the lumen of an adjoining segment (intussuscipiens). Intussusception most often occurs in young children, and most are ileocolic (see Chapter 7). Most intussusceptions that involve only the small bowel are ileoileal and are idiopathic (Fig. 6–30). Idiopathic intussusception probably occurs from hypertrophied lymphoid tissue from a preceding viral infection. Infrequently, intussusceptions have a discernible lead point, such as a Meckel diverticulum, lymphoma, duplication cyst, or polyp.

Trauma to the small bowel can be difficult to detect radiologically and often is suggested by unexplained mesenteric or free intraperitoneal fluid seen on CT. Mass effect from mural hematomas can cause luminal narrowing (Fig. 6–31).

Suggested Readings

Antes G, Eggemann F: Small Bowel Radiology: Introduction and Atlas. New York, Springer-Verlag, 1986.

Chen MYM, Zagoria RJ, Ott DJ, Gelfand DW: Radiology of the Small Bowel. New York, Igaku-Shoin, 1992.

Gore RM, Levine MS, Laufer I: Textbook of Gastrointestinal Radiology, 2nd ed. Philadelphia, WB Saunders, 2000.

Herlinger H, Maglinte D: Clinical Radiology of the Small Intestine. Philadelphia, WB Saunders, 1989.

Houston JD, Davis M: Fundamentals of Fluoroscopy. Philadelphia, WB Saunders, 2001.

Marshak RH, Lindner AE: Radiology of the Small Intestine, 2nd ed. Philadelphia, WB Saunders, 1976.

SEVEN

Large Intestine

MICHAEL DAVIS, M.D., AND JEFFREY D. HOUSTON, M.D.

Normal Anatomy

The **large intestine** is about 1.5 m in length and is divided into the cecum, appendix, colon (ascending, transverse, descending, and sigmoid), and rectum (Fig. 7–1). Distinguishing characteristics of the large intestine include three longitudinally oriented bands of muscle (taeniae coli), sacculations (haustra), and fat-filled pouches of omentum (epiploic appendages).

The most proximal portion of the large intestine is the **cecum,** which is normally located in the right lower quadrant and communicates medially with the terminal ileum through the ileocecal valve. The cecum measures 5 to 7 cm in length and usually is enveloped by peritoneum and anchored to the posterior abdominal wall.

The **vermiform appendix** is a wormlike tubular structure that is contiguous with the inferior cecum. It averages 8 cm in length and can be located in a variety of positions: retrocecal, pelvic, or retrocolic. The appendix is considered to be a vestigial organ in humans but has immunologic functions because of the lymphoid tissue that it contains.

The **ascending colon** extends superiorly from the cecum on the right side of the abdomen. It is covered by peritoneum, which affixes it to the posterior abdominal wall. The segment of the ascending colon that courses to the left and around the liver is termed the **hepatic flexure.** Interposition of the hepatic flexure between the dome of the liver and the right hemidiaphragm, termed the **Chilaiditi sign,** can be a normal variant (Fig. 7–2).

Crossing the abdomen from right to left, the **transverse colon** is a mobile segment of colon that is attached to the posterior abdominal wall by a mesentery. This segment occasionally can droop into the pelvis and is described as being ptotic.

The **descending colon** extends inferiorly from the **splenic flexure** on the left side of the abdomen. It is usually retroperitoneal but occasionally has a mesentery.

As suggested by its name (from the Greek letter *sigma*), the **sigmoid colon** has an S-shaped configuration. It lies deep in the pelvis and usually has a long mesentery. The sigmoid colon can be tortuous, especially in older individuals.

The **rectum** (from the Latin word *rectus,*

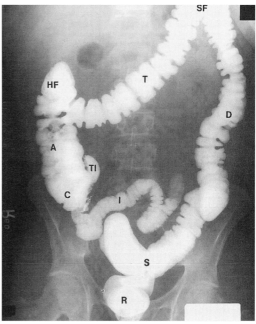

Figure 7–1. Normal anatomy of the large intestine. Single-contrast barium enema allows visualization of the segments of the large intestine and distal small bowel: ileum (I), terminal ileum (TI), cecum (C), ascending colon (A), hepatic flexure (HF), transverse colon (T), splenic flexure (SF), descending colon (D), sigmoid colon (S), rectum (R). (From Houston JD, Davis M: Fundamentals of Fluoroscopy. Philadelphia, WB Saunders, 2001.)

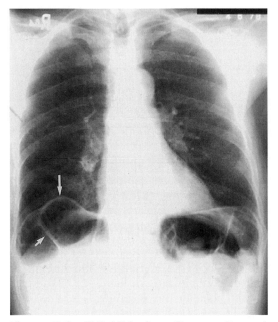

Figure 7–2. Chilaiditi sign. Chest radiograph demonstrates interposition of the hepatic flexure between the liver and the right hemidiaphragm (Chilaiditi sign) *(large arrow)* in a patient with chronic vague abdominal pain. Note the colonic haustral fold *(small arrow)*.

meaning "straight") is the terminal portion of the large intestine. It is fixed in location and has no mesentery. The rectum is continuous with the anal canal distally.

The **colon** technically refers to the portion of the large intestine that extends between the cecum and rectum. The term commonly (although inaccurately) is used as a synonym for the entire large intestine.

Imaging Modalities

Common indications that warrant radiologic examination of the large intestine include abdominal pain, obstruction, bleeding, colonic infection, diarrhea, constipation, abdominal masses, and personal or family history of colon cancer or polyps. Screening examinations for colon carcinoma or precancerous polyps are performed commonly in individuals older than age 50.

Radiologic evaluation by contrast enema has proved to be a useful method for the evaluation of large bowel abnormalities. Fluoroscopic procedures comprise most radiologic examinations of the colon. Examination of the large intestine can be performed using single-contrast or double-contrast technique. For most routine examinations, patients are required to undergo a bowel preparation on the day preceding the examination to cleanse the bowel of residual fecal material that could obscure underlying pathology.

Single-contrast barium enema requires filling the entire large intestine with a low-density (15% to 20% weight volume [w/v]) barium suspension, while images of each segment are obtained (Fig. 7–3). This method easily shows diverticular disease, masses greater than 1 cm, strictures, extrinsic masses, malrotation, and advanced inflammatory and infectious disease.

Water-soluble contrast enema using iodinated contrast may be used to evaluate the large intestine in a manner similar to the single-contrast barium enema. This examination can be performed safely when there is suspicion of bowel perforation. Because of the hyperosmotic effect of the iodinated contrast, this method has an additional use of having a therapeutic effect on colonic pseudo-obstruction and impaction.

In a **double-contrast barium enema,** the bowel is paralyzed temporarily with systemically administered glucagon, filled with 350 mL of dense barium (200% to 250% w/v), and insufflated with air. Images are obtained as the patient rolls into various positions to coat the mucosa with dense barium (Fig. 7–4). This examination requires meticulous radiographic technique and significant patient cooperation. Patients that have significantly decreased mobility or are unable to retain the insufflated air are imaged best with single-contrast technique. Double-contrast technique is best for evaluating subtle mucosal disease, including early inflammatory or infectious processes and polyps less than 1 cm in size.

Dynamic proctography is an uncommonly performed study used to evaluate patients who have difficulty defecating. The rectum is filled with barium paste, and the patient is placed on a radiolucent commode (Brunswick chair). Images are obtained while the patient performs various evacuation maneuvers.

Measurement of colonic transit can be performed by having the patient ingest a capsule containing a predetermined quantity of radiopaque rings. Delayed abdominal radiographs can be used to quantify the

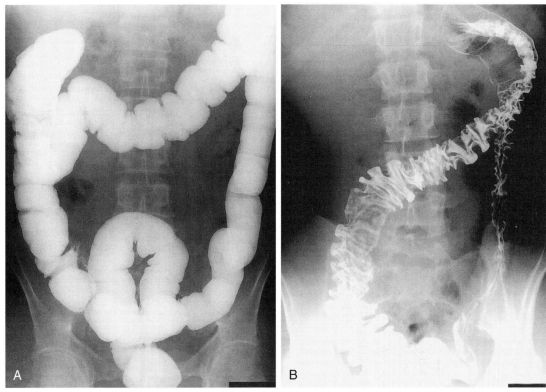

Figure 7–3. Normal single-contrast barium enema. Anteroposterior full column **(A)** and postevacuation **(B)** images from a single-contrast barium enema. Use of a proper barium suspension and correct technical factors permit the ability to see faintly through the barium column.

number of retained rings as an indicator of motility.

Computed tomography (CT) of the colon has limited applications. It often is used for further evaluation of established abnormalities, such as for assessing extramural extension of malignancy. CT is used routinely as a primary imaging modality for appendicitis and diverticulitis. Imaging can be optimized by filling the colon with dilute contrast agent immediately before scanning.

Ultrasound can be used for diagnosis of appendicitis and intussusception, particularly in children. **Nuclear medicine imaging** is used to localize the site of gastrointestinal hemorrhage because only active bleeding can be visualized with **angiography.**

Functional Abnormalities

Meconium plug syndrome is a condition that occurs in the full-term neonate in which a plug of thickened meconium becomes lodged in the colon and causes obstruction. This condition is thought to be precipitated by poor peristalsis from neuronal underdevelopment. The distal colon is usually of normal caliber.

Colonic pseudo-obstruction (Ogilvie syndrome) is an ailment that often exhibits marked colonic distention but lacks mechanical obstruction (Fig. 7–5). This syndrome occurs most often in elderly patients. A water-soluble contrast enema can be diagnostic and therapeutic.

Structural Abnormalities

Congenital abnormalities include microcolon, duplication, atresia, and imperforate anus. **Microcolon** results from a distal obstruction that prohibits sufficient succus entericus from reaching the distal colonic segments (Fig. 7–6). **Colonic duplication** is a rare abnormality of recanalization in which colonic segments or the entire colon can be duplicated (Fig. 7–7). **Colonic atresia** and **stenosis** are rare and are believed to result from an intrauterine vascular insult. **Imperforate anus** is a relatively common condition

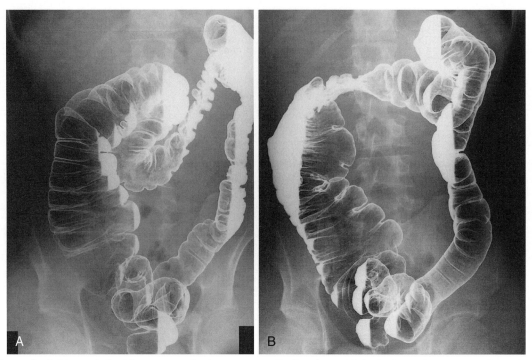

Figure 7–4. Normal double-contrast barium enema. Right **(A)** and left **(B)** lateral decubitus films from a double-contrast barium enema reveal how subtle mucosal detail can be visualized when coated properly with dense barium and with sufficient gaseous distention of the lumen. The narrowed areas represent collapse of nondistended segments.

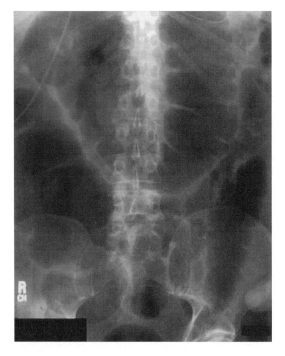

Figure 7–5. Ogilvie syndrome. Conventional radiograph of the abdomen demonstrates diffuse gaseous distention of the colon.

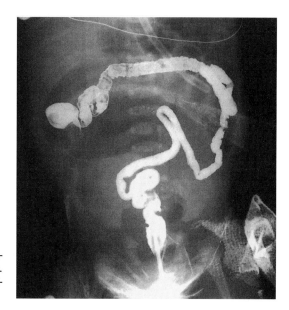

Figure 7–6. Microcolon. Single-contrast barium enema illustrates diminished caliber of the colon. (From Williamson SL: Essentials of Pediatric Radiology. Philadelphia, WB Saunders, 2001.)

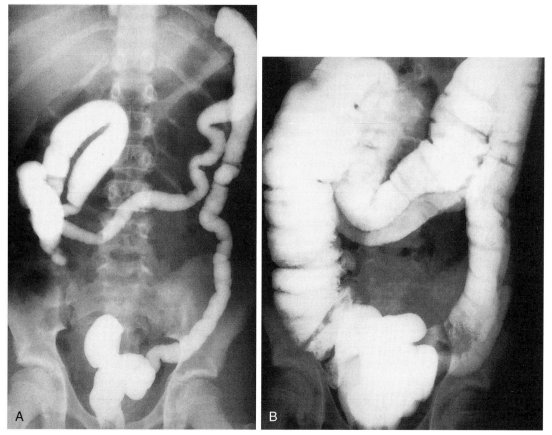

Figure 7–7. Colonic duplication. A and **B,** Sequential images from a single-contrast barium enema show filling of a small-caliber colon (the duplication), followed by filling of a larger caliber second channel in a patient with complete colonic duplication.

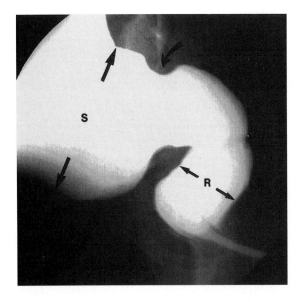

Figure 7–8. Hirschsprung disease. Single-contrast water-soluble enema shows a normal caliber rectum (R) in contrast to the increased diameter of the sigmoid colon (S). A transitional zone *(curved arrow)* demarcates the abrupt transition from normal to abnormal innervation. (From Houston JD, Davis M: Fundamentals of Fluoroscopy. Philadelphia, WB Saunders, 2001.)

that is associated with spinal and urinary abnormalities. Fistulas to the skin, urinary tract, or other adjacent structures can occur with anorectal malformations.

Hirschsprung disease (congenital aganglionic megacolon) is a congenital condition in which there is arrested migration of neural crest cells, which leaves a segment lacking ganglion cells. This disease occurs in about 1 out of 5000 live births with a 4:1 male predominance. Radiographically a transitional zone is apparent on contrast enemas, and there is proximal dilation of the colon (megacolon) (Fig. 7–8).

Abnormalities of rotation of the midgut during embryologic development can result in a variety of anomalous configurations of the colon (Fig. 7–9). In **colonic nonrotation,**

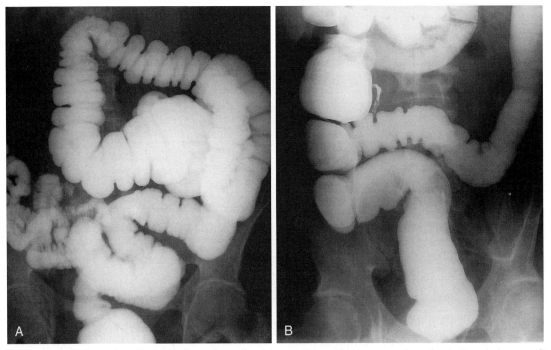

Figure 7–9. Malrotation. Two single-contrast barium enemas exhibit examples of rotational abnormalities of the colon: **A,** The colon lies almost entirely in the left abdomen. **B,** The sigmoid colon is abnormally located in the right lower quadrant.

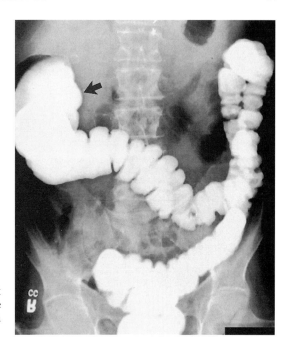

Figure 7–10. Subhepatic cecum. Single-contrast barium enema reveals subhepatic placement of the cecum *(arrow)* instead of in the normal position in the right lower quadrant.

the colon is located in the left abdomen, whereas partial rotational abnormalities are termed **colonic malrotation** and can produce a spectrum of abnormal positions. There is no correlation, however, between rotation and the descent of the cecum into the right lower quadrant. As the colon grows, the cecum normally is forced into the right lower quadrant. An undescended cecum results from failure of late colonic growth (Fig. 7–10).

Abnormalities of fixation to the posterior abdominal wall permit mobility of colonic segments, which can be asymptomatic or predispose to herniation or volvulus. A mobile segment can herniate into any potential space, such as the lesser peritoneal sac, defects in the abdominal wall, femoral space, or inguinal canal (Fig. 7–11).

A **mobile cecum** refers to nonfixation of the cecum to the posterior abdominal wall. This anomaly allows for potential volvulus of the cecum and ascending colon. The right colon can be located anywhere in the abdomen, including interposed between the liver and the right hemidiaphragm. A mobile cecum or ascending colon can herniate into femoral or inguinoscrotal hernia sacs.

Cecal volvulus is a surgical emergency that can have a high mortality rate because of vascular occlusion and rapidly ensuing infarction. The most common form of cecal volvulus is axial torsion, in which the cecum

is twisted around the longitudinal axis of the ascending colon (organoaxial) (Fig. 7–12*A*). The distended cecum can be situated anywhere in the abdomen, but often is in the midabdomen or left upper quadrant. On contrast enema examination, there is a beaklike appearance at the site of torsion (Fig. 7–12*B*). **Cecal bascule** is another form of volvulus in which the cecum flips anteromedially to occupy a transverse orientation in the abdomen (mesentericoaxial) (Fig. 7–12*C*).

Sigmoid volvulus is one of the most common forms of gastrointestinal volvulus. Similar to cecal volvulus, it can be a serious condition. In many cases, diagnosis can be made on the basis of conventional radiographs that reveal marked gaseous distention of the sigmoid colon, which appears to rise out of the pelvis (Fig. 7–13*A*). On contrast enema examination, there is a classic beaklike appearance at the site of torsion (Fig. 7–13*B*).

Diverticula are frequently seen structural abnormalities of the colon whose complications comprise a large percentage of colonic disease. A complete discussion of diverticular disease follows.

Diverticular Disease

Colonic diverticulosis is a common finding that increases with age. These pulsion

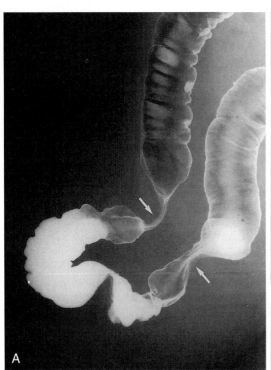

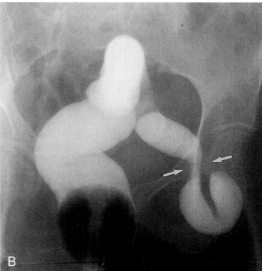

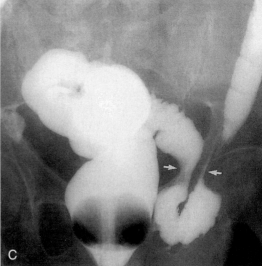

Figure 7–11. Colonic herniations. Multiple barium enemas exhibit varieties of colonic herniations (*arrows* indicate hernia necks): **A,** Extension of the sigmoid colon through a ventral hernia. **B,** Herniation of the sigmoid colon into the left femoral space. **C,** Herniation of the sigmoid colon into the left inguinal canal.

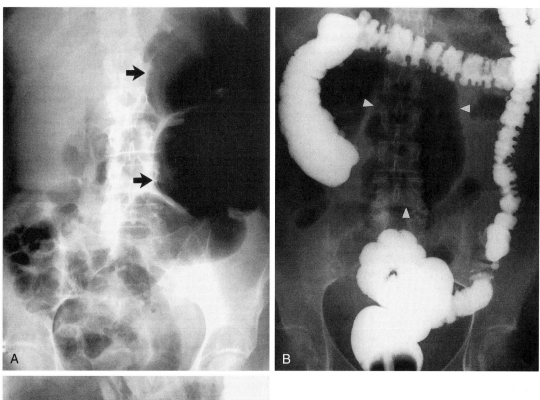

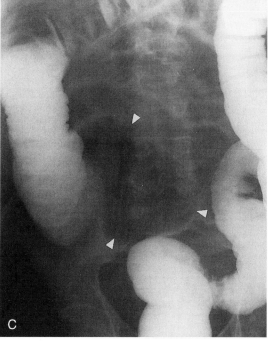

Figure 7–12. Cecal volvulus. A, Conventional radiograph demonstrates a large gas-filled structure in the left upper quadrant *(arrows)*, which is suspicious for cecal volvulus. **B,** Single-contrast barium enema confirms cecal volvulus by lack of filling of the abnormally located cecum *(arrowheads)*. **C,** Single-contrast barium enema shows that the cecum has flipped anteromedially to occupy a transverse orientation in the abdomen, creating a cecal bascule *(arrowheads)*.

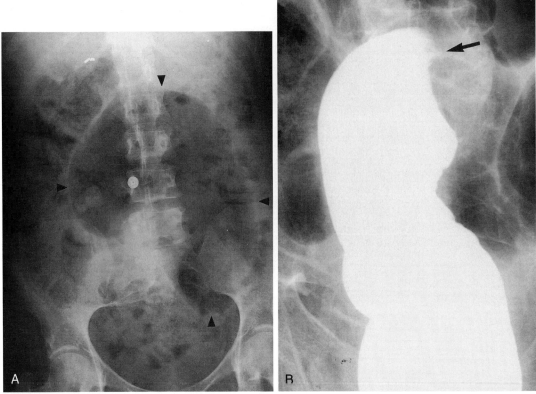

Figure 7–13. Sigmoid volvulus. A, Conventional radiograph reveals a distended loop of gas-filled bowel *(arrowheads)* ascending from the pelvis, suggesting sigmoid volvulus. **B,** Single-contrast barium enema shows filling of the rectum and distal sigmoid, with abrupt beaklike termination at the site of volvulus *(arrow).*

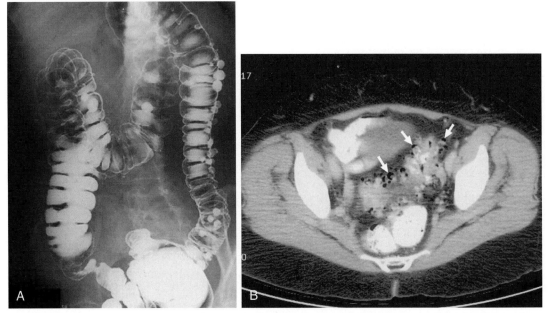

Figure 7–14. Colonic diverticulosis. A, Double-contrast barium enema displays multiple outpouchings of the colonic wall in a patient with severe diverticulosis. **B,** Peripheral rounded lucencies *(arrows)* represent collections of air located in sigmoid diverticula, as seen on CT with rectal contrast.

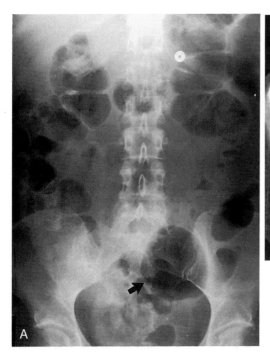

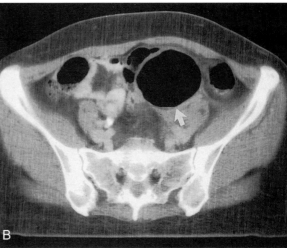

Figure 7–15. Giant sigmoid diverticulum. A, Conventional abdominal radiograph indicates a large rounded lucency *(arrow)* in the expected area of the sigmoid colon. **B,** CT confirms the diagnosis of a giant sigmoid diverticulum *(arrow).*

diverticula are thought to be caused by insufficient dietary fiber, leading to increased intraluminal pressure and protrusion of mucosa through anatomic areas of weakness in the muscular wall of the colon (Fig. 7–14). Single diverticula may be seen in patients as young as 30 years old, and hundreds of diverticula may be evident in elderly patients. The most common site of diverticulum formation is the sigmoid colon, but isolated diverticula may be seen in other segments of the colon, including the cecum.

Another variation of diverticulosis is the **giant diverticulum,** which nearly always occurs in the sigmoid colon. These thick-walled diverticula have no mucosal lining and connect to the colon through a tiny orifice (Fig. 7–15), which may prohibit filling during a contrast enema.

Although *diverticulosis* refers to the presence of diverticula, *diverticulitis* indicates diverticular inflammation (Fig. 7–16). Bleeding from erosion into mural arteries, perforation, and abscess formation are the most common complications. CT examination can identify intramural and pericolic abscesses, pericolic sinus tracts, or fistula formation to other organs. Fistulas may form to loops of small bowel, ureter, bladder, vagina, skin, retroperitoneum, hip, and thigh. Colovesical fistulas are more common in men, whereas women can have colovaginal fistulas.

Appendicitis

Acute appendicitis generally is seen in adolescents and young adults but can occur in patients of any age. Despite its prevalence, appendicitis can be sometimes difficult to diagnose clinically. Because many conditions can mimic the signs and symptoms of

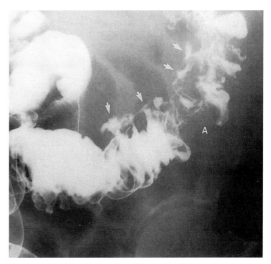

Figure 7–16. Colonic diverticulitis. Single-contrast barium enema shows diffuse spasticity, perforation of a sigmoid diverticulum with intramural fistulas *(arrows),* and an intramural abscess (A).

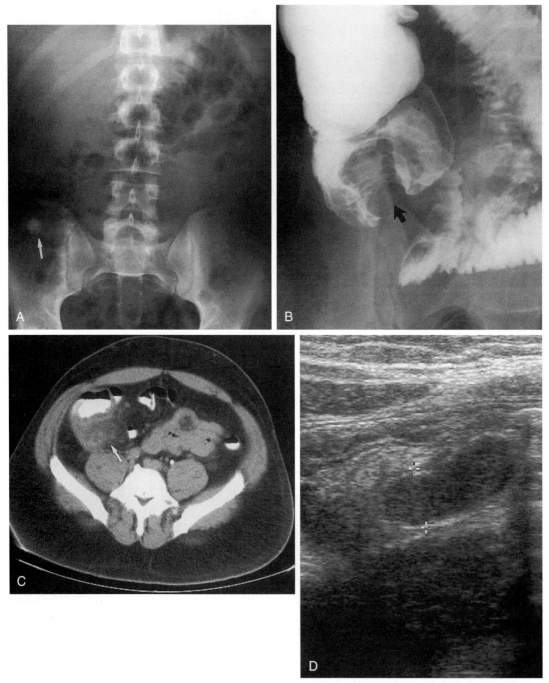

Figure 7–17. Appendicitis. Various imaging modalities demonstrate findings of appendicitis: **A,** Conventional radiograph shows a calcified appendicolith *(arrow)*. **B,** Single-contrast barium enema shows deformity of the cecum from an inflamed appendix *(arrow)*. **C,** Inflammatory changes surround the appendix on CT. **D,** Ultrasound reveals a noncompressible tubular structure (between calipers) in the right lower quadrant, representing a dilated appendix. (**D,** From Williamson SL: Essentials of Pediatric Radiology. Philadelphia, WB Saunders, 2001.)

appendicitis, imaging is often requested to confirm the diagnosis (Fig. 7–17). Appendicitis is associated with mechanical obstruction of a portion of the appendiceal lumen, often because of a fecalith (appendicolith). Continued secretion of fluid into the obstructed appendix results in distention and vascular compression. Ischemia, bacterial proliferation, gangrene, and perforation complicate the condition. Periappendiceal abscesses may occur.

Radiographic findings in appendicitis include a right lower quadrant localized ileus, splinting of the lumbosacral spine, obliteration of the psoas shadow and properitoneal fat line, abnormal gas collections in the right lower quadrant, a mass, a radiopaque appendicolith (10%), and occasionally air within the appendix. Pericecal inflammatory changes and appendiceal dilation may be evident with CT. On ultrasound, appendicitis is diagnosed when a noncompressible tubular structure with a thickness greater than 6 mm is located in the right lower quadrant.

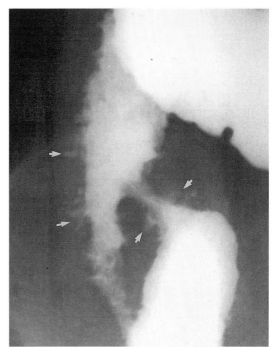

Figure 7–18. Colonic tuberculosis. Single-contrast barium enema displays a narrowed terminal ileum and "coned" cecum, as well as multiple small ulcerations *(arrows)*.

Infectious Colitis

Pathogens that cause infectious colitis include a wide range of bacterial, parasitic, fungal, and viral agents. **Salmonellosis** and **shigellosis** (bacillary dysentery) acutely cause patchy areas of deep ulcerations with inflammation and thickening of the wall, which can lead to scarring and fibrosis. Salmonellosis occurs mostly as a pancolitis, whereas shigellosis preferentially involves the left colon.

Colonic tuberculosis usually has a segmental distribution and favors the ileocecal region. Ulcerations of varying depths and luminal narrowing are seen (Fig. 7–18). Differentiation from Crohn disease can be difficult, with both diseases featuring "skip lesions." Only about half of patients with colonic tuberculosis have an abnormal chest radiograph.

Antibiotic-associated colitis (pseudomembranous colitis) classically is caused by toxins from overgrowth of *Clostridium difficile,* a normal colonic microbe. Overgrowth can be precipitated by antibiotic, steroid, or chemotherapy administration. This disease is characterized by formation of an adherent inflammatory **pseudomembrane,** which is a plaquelike coagulum of denuded epithelium, inflammatory cells, and mucus, which may

be apparent radiologically. The pseudomembrane is not specific for antibiotic-associated colitis and can be seen in any type of colitis that results in severe mucosal injury. Bowel wall thickening, "thumbprinting," and pneumatosis also may occur (Fig. 7–19).

Amebiasis (amebic dysentery), caused by the protozoan *Entamoeba histolytica,* is manifested radiographically by superficial ulceration and may be difficult to differentiate from ulcerative colitis. The cecum is involved in 90% of cases, with scattered areas of involvement in the remainder of the colon, particularly in the flexures and rectosigmoid (Fig. 7–20). In the late stages of the disease, the cecum narrows and appears cone-shaped. Amebiasis can form an **ameboma,** an inflammatory mass that may simulate a carcinoma. Amebiasis also mimics Crohn disease with skip lesions.

Although **Chagas disease** is encountered rarely in the United States, infection with the protozoan *Trypanosoma cruzi* remains an important cause of infectious colitis in other regions of the world. Greatest morbidity originates from the heart, but the esophagus and colon also are common sites of involvement. The trypanosomes invade the bowel

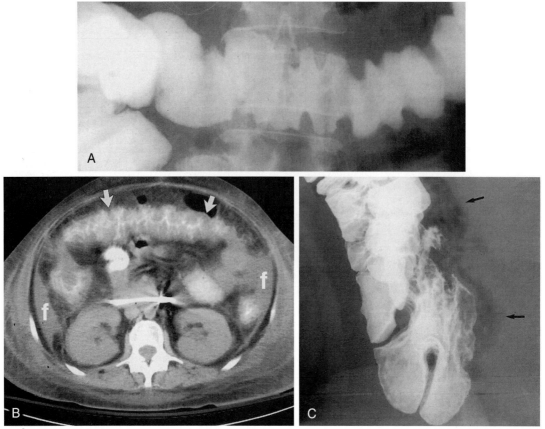

Figure 7–19. Antibiotic-associated colitis. A, Single-contrast barium enema displays narrowing and subtle "thumbprinting" of the transverse colon. **B,** Abdominal CT in another patient illustrates marked thickening of the transverse colon *(arrows)* as well as free intraperitoneal fluid (f) in the paracolic gutters. **C,** Single-contrast barium enema in a third patient helps to diagnose intramural air *(arrows),* representing pneumatosis intestinalis that has arisen as a complication from antibiotic-associated colitis.

wall and destroy the ganglion cells of the enteric plexus. After the acute phase, chronic disease may persist for decades and can be one of the causes of **acquired megacolon.** The colon becomes aperistaltic, dilated, and distended with fecal material.

Cytomegalovirus colitis is associated with immunosuppression, particularly acquired immunodeficiency syndrome. Early radiographic findings include mucosal granularity and ulcerations. Other opportunistic colonic infections include *Mycobacterium avium-intracellulare, C. difficile,* and *Cryptosporidium.*

Amebiasis, tuberculosis, and actinomycosis tend to involve the cecal area, ultimately forming a "coned" cecum. Tuberculosis and actinomycosis tend to involve the terminal ileum, whereas amebiasis rarely does. Yersiniosis has the appearance of Crohn dis-

ease in the terminal ileum but does not cause fistula formation or strictures. *Campylobacter* colitis and *C. difficile* infection can have a radiographic appearance that may be indistinguishable from ulcerative colitis. Amebiasis and tuberculosis may mimic Crohn disease in their ability to form skip lesions anywhere in the colon.

Sexually transmitted diseases, such as condylomata acuminata, lymphogranuloma venereum (serovars of *Chlamydia trachomatis*), and gonorrhea may affect the anus and rectum, inciting edema, ulcers, and strictures.

Inflammatory Bowel Disease

Idiopathic inflammatory bowel disease is a collective term for Crohn disease and ul-

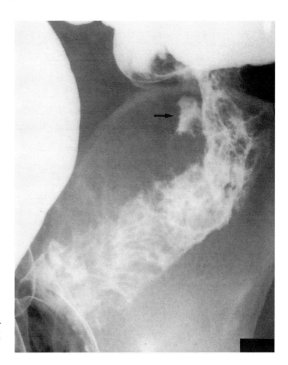

Figure 7–20. Amebiasis. Single-contrast barium enema demonstrates severe mucosal irregularity and ulceration *(arrow)* in the sigmoid colon.

cerative colitis, two inflammatory diseases of unknown cause. These two chronic and relapsing diseases share many characteristics and often are discussed together.

Ulcerative colitis is a mucosal inflammatory process that begins in the rectum and progresses retrograde, involving varying lengths or the entire colon. The most common clinical findings are rectal bleeding, abdominal pain, and diarrhea. The greatest incidence of onset is at about 20 years of age.

Barium enema best shows the range of mucosal abnormalities seen in ulcerative colitis (Fig. 7–21). In the early stages of affliction, the mucosa is characterized as having a granular, velvet-like, or sandlike appearance. The disease begins in the distal rectum and progresses retrograde with uniform involvement of the mucosa. As the disease advances, ulcers of varying size and depth begin to occur. The ulcers have been characterized as "collar button" or flasklike, the appearance representing undermining of the ulcer bed. During severe active disease, the mucosa can be denuded by the intense inflammatory reaction, sparing small islands of mucosa and submucosa that are referred to as **inflammatory pseudopolyps.** As healing occurs and mucosal cells regenerate, areas of aggressive regeneration may produce **postinflammatory polyps;** tiny finger-like projections of mucosa are referred to as **filiform polyps.**

The terminal ileum can be affected in patients with pancolitis. The ileocecal valve becomes patulous, and inflammatory changes are seen in the ileum that consist of luminal widening and mucosal effacement. Some controversy exists as to whether this represents *backwash ileitis* or whether the disease primarily is involving the distal ileum. On healing of the inflammatory process, residual changes other than postinflammatory pseudopolyps include shortening of the colon, luminal narrowing, loss of haustral folds, and widening of the presacral space.

Toxic megacolon can occur in several inflammatory and infectious diseases of the colon, particularly in ulcerative colitis. This severe, life-threatening condition is a result of a massive and extensive inflammatory process that affects the deep tissues of the colonic wall with loss of integrity of the supporting structures. The colon becomes markedly dilated, and the walls become thickened and edematous (Fig. 7–22).

Carcinoma is a well-known complication of ulcerative colitis. The risk of cancer increases after the first decade and increases significantly in patients with pancolitis. Carcinoma arises in dysplastic epithelium in ul-

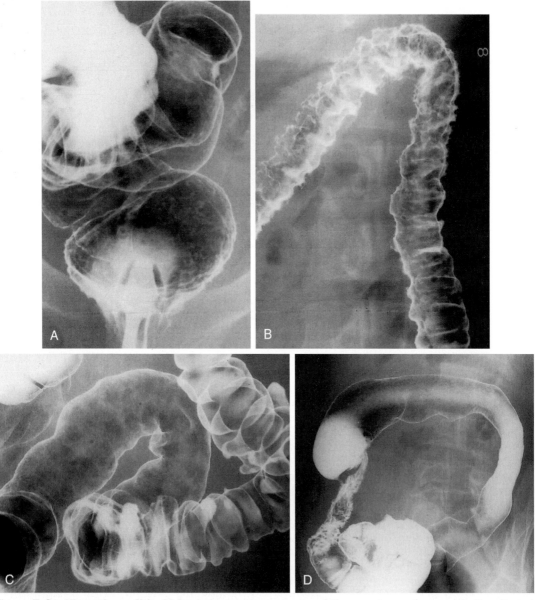

Figure 7–21. Ulcerative colitis. Multiple barium enemas reveal the spectrum of mucosal alterations in patients with ulcerative colitis: **A,** Mild mucosal nodularity of the rectum. **B,** Severe mucosal irregularity of the splenic flexure with small ulcerations. **C,** Focal absence of mucosal features and haustra in a segment of the sigmoid colon. **D,** Diffuse obliteration of mucosal features and haustra with foreshortening from chronic ulcerative colitis.

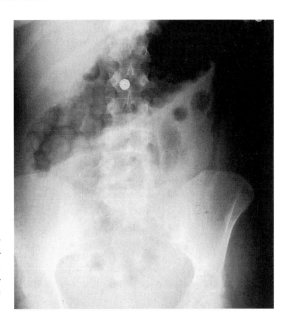

Figure 7–22. Toxic megacolon. Conventional abdominal radiograph shows dilation of the transverse colon, which contains multiple rounded opacities representing inflammatory pseudopolyps. This occurred as a complication of ulcerative colitis.

cerative colitis, as opposed to arising in adenomas. Cancer surveillance with long-term ulcerative colitis is done primarily by colonoscopy with biopsy.

Liver (hepatitis), biliary tract (sclerosing cholangitis, cholangiocarcinoma), and skeletal (sacroileitis, ankylosing spondylitis) sequelae of ulcerative colitis are well known. The eyes, skin, kidneys, and lungs may also be affected.

When initially described in 1932, **Crohn disease** (regional enteritis) was thought to be confined to the terminal ileum and was named *terminal ileitis.* The pathologic hallmark of Crohn disease is the presence of noncaseating granulomas. The cause of Crohn disease remains an enigma, although diet, genetics, antibiotics, smoking, oral contraceptives, measles infection in early childhood, tuberculosis, bacterial antigens, viral infections, and abnormal mesenteric blood supply (granulomatous vasculitis) all have been proposed as possible causes. A multifactorial cause in which hereditary and environmental factors interact to produce the disease is likely.

Barium enema best shows the range of mucosal abnormalities seen in Crohn disease (Fig. 7–23). The progression of findings begins with nodular lymphoid hyperplasia and superficial **aphthous ulcerations,** with normal intervening mucosa. As the disease progresses, the bowel wall becomes thickened. Deeper ulcerations occur, and deep transverse and horizontal fissuring gives a coarse **"cobblestone"** appearance to the mucosa. Areas of asymmetry, where one side of the bowel is more involved than the other, and **skip lesions,** in which areas of involvement are interspersed between normal areas of mucosa, are characteristic findings. Later changes include deep fissures that have a **"rose-thorn"** appearance in profile, fistula or sinus tract formation, widening of the presacral space, and pericolonic abscess formation. After healing occurs, postinflammatory polyp formation (including filiform polyp) is possible.

Any segment of the gastrointestinal tract, from the mouth to the rectum, can be involved. The terminal ileum and right colon are involved most commonly. Isolated colonic involvement and isolated small intestinal involvement occur less frequently. Extraintestinal associations of Crohn disease include arthritides, erythema nodosum, uveitis, and cholangitis. Although cholangiocarcinoma is seen commonly in ulcerative colitis, it is rare in Crohn disease.

Other Colitides

Immunosuppressed patients, particularly patients undergoing chemotherapy, are at risk for developing **typhlitis** (neutropenic colitis), an acute necrotizing colitis of unknown pathogenesis that involves the pericecal region. Symptoms may mimic appendiceal abscess. The diagnosis usually is made by ex-

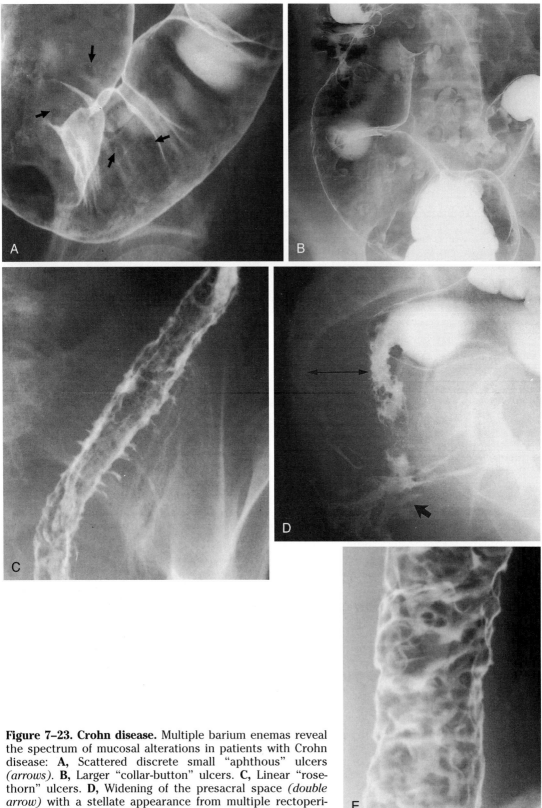

Figure 7–23. Crohn disease. Multiple barium enemas reveal
the spectrum of mucosal alterations in patients with Crohn
disease: **A,** Scattered discrete small "aphthous" ulcers
(arrows). **B,** Larger "collar-button" ulcers. **C,** Linear "rose-
thorn" ulcers. **D,** Widening of the presacral space *(double
arrow)* with a stellate appearance from multiple rectoperi-
neal fistulas *(large arrow)*. **E,** "Cobblestone" mucosa.

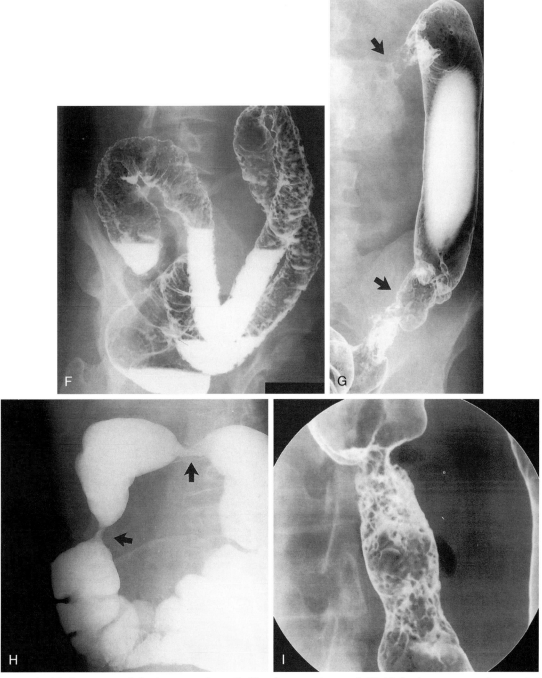

Figure 7–23 *Continued.* **F,** Crohn pancolitis. **G,** Skip lesions *(arrows).* **H,** Multiple strictures *(arrows).* **I,** Postinflammatory polyps.

cluding the usual causes of inflammation and infection and considering the patient's immunosupressed state. Radiographic findings include thickening of the cecum and pericecal inflammatory changes (Fig. 7–24).

Ischemic colitis mimics ulcerative colitis and Crohn disease. Causes are vasculitis, atherosclerosis, embolism, venous thrombosis, a low-flow state from cardiac disease, and drug abuse (such as intravenous methamphetamine). A classic radiographic finding is thumbprinting, principally in the

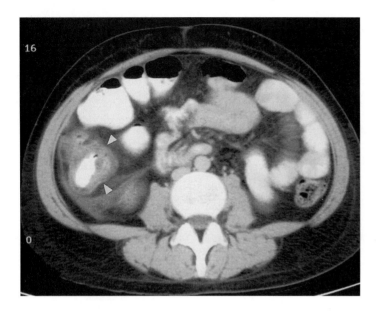

Figure 7–24. Typhlitis. Diffuse thickening of the cecum and adjacent free intraperitoneal fluid in the right paracolic gutter is seen on abdominal CT with rectal contrast, representing typhlitis in a leukemic patient.

splenic flexure, left colon, or sigmoid colon (Fig. 7–25), although any segment of the colon may be involved. Mucosal irregularity, followed by ulcerations, can develop a pattern similar to ulcerative colitis. Healing can occur with a return of the lumen to normal, or the disease can progress to gangrene, perforation, and death. Segmental strictures of the colon may result from ischemia.

Necrotizing enterocolitis occurs most commonly in premature neonates. It is associated with hypoxia, hypotension, stress,

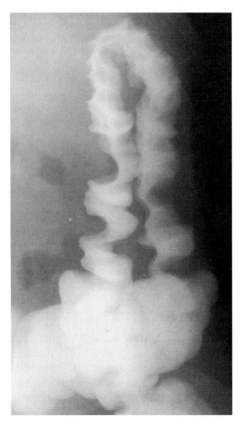

Figure 7–25. Ischemic colitis. Single-contrast barium enema shows narrowing and "thumbprinting" of the splenic flexure. The splenic flexure is a particularly vulnerable colonic segment for ischemia because it is in a watershed region of two vascular territories.

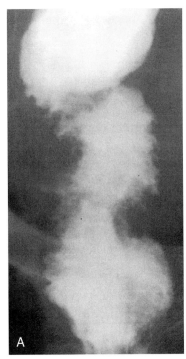

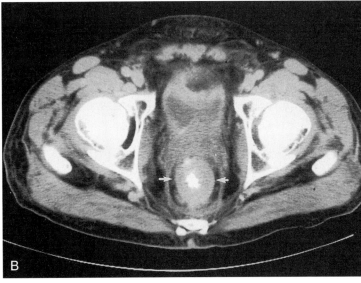

Figure 7–26. Radiation proctitis. The effects of radiation, as seen by single-contrast barium enema **(A)** and pelvic CT **(B)**, are similar to ischemic colitis, including edema and ulceration, which are followed by eventual fibrosis and stenosis. Note the mural thickening and lumenal narrowing in the rectum *(arrows)*.

and infection. The cause is most likely multifactorial, but involves ischemia and mucosal breakdown that permits pneumatosis and infection. The most commonly affected segments of bowel are the distal ileum and ascending colon. Radiographic findings include ileus and linear or bubbly pneumatosis. Complications are perforation, sepsis, and stricture.

Radiation colitis is essentially an ischemic vasculitis following radiation therapy and presenting 6 months to 2 years after treatment. Acute changes may simulate ulcerative colitis and ischemic or infectious colitis with short or long strictures (Fig. 7–26).

Benign Neoplasms

Double-contrast examinations occasionally reveal **lymphoid hyperplasia,** which simply refers to enlarged lymphoid follicles on the mucosal surface (Fig. 7–27). The clinical significance of these lesions is unknown, although they are thought to represent reactive change from inflammation. They can be seen in asymptomatic patients, however.

A **polyp** is a growth that protrudes from a mucous membrane. Three types of polyps can be encountered: hyperplastic, adenomatous, and hamartomatous. Polyps may be either pedunculated (stalked) or sessile

(flat). **Hyperplastic polyps** (pseudopolyps) represent the majority of polyps arising in the large intestine. They are not true polyps, but rather represent protrusions of mucosa

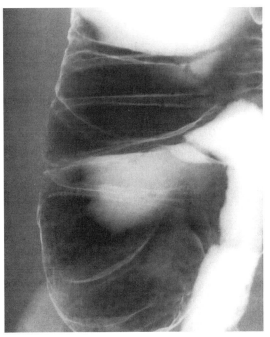

Figure 7–27. Lymphoid hyperplasia. Double-contrast barium enema allows faint visualization of tiny nodules of hyperplastic lymphoid follicles in the cecum.

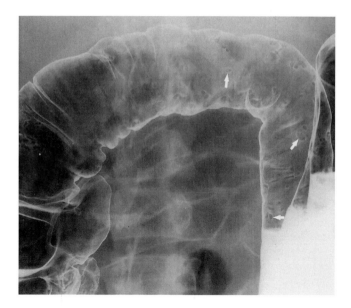

Figure 7–28. Postinflammatory pseudopolyps. Small scattered finger-like projections of mucosa *(arrows)* are visualized in the transverse colon with double-contrast barium enema.

that resemble a polyp because of surrounding mucosal damage. They may occur throughout the colon but are seen most commonly in the rectum and sigmoid segments. They are usually 5 mm or less in diameter and occur in chronic inflammatory conditions (Fig. 7–28). These polyps have virtually no malignant potential.

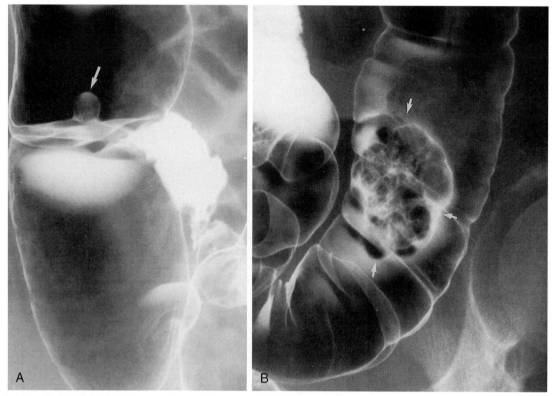

Figure 7–29. Adenomatous polyps. Double-contrast barium enemas reveal a small polyp *(arrow)* at the junction of the cecum and ascending colon **(A),** and a villous adenoma *(arrows)* in the distal descending colon **(B).**

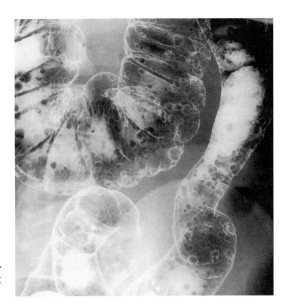

Figure 7–30. Familial adenomatous polyposis syndrome. Thousands of adenomatous polyps carpet the colon.

Adenomatous polyps represent 25% of colonic polyps and are true neoplasms. An **adenoma** is a neoplasm that arises from intestinal epithelium; most adenomas grow toward the lumen (Fig. 7–29). The size of polyps can vary from less than 5 mm to several centimeters in diameter. Adenomas may be solitary or multiple or may carpet the mucosa extensively, as in the polyposis syndromes. Adenomatous lesions arise from epithelial dysplasia, which ranges from mild to severe dysplasia that constitutes carcinoma in situ. Most (if not all) cases of colon carcinoma are thought to arise from adenomatous polyps, with the exception of dysplastic mucosa in ulcerative colitis.

Hamartomatous polyps represent focal hamartomatous malformations of the mucosa that do not have malignant potential. **Juvenile polyps** are large (1 to 3 cm diameter), smooth hamartomas that occur sporadically in children or can be seen in the rare **juvenile polyposis syndrome.** Most juvenile polyps are seen in children younger than 5 years of age. Isolated smaller hamartomatous polyps found in adults are termed **retention polyps.** Large pedunculated polyps are seen in **Peutz-Jeghers syndrome,** a rare condition characterized by the widespread presence of hamartomatous polyps. These patients have a high risk of developing carcinoma from concomitant adenomatous neoplasms.

Familial polyposis syndromes are uncommon hereditary conditions that are divided into Peutz-Jeghers syndrome (hamartomatous polyps) and familial adenomatous polyposis (adenomatous polyps). **Familial adenomatous polyposis** is characterized by carpeting of the mucosa by hundreds to thousands of adenomas (Fig. 7–30). **Gardner syndrome** is a variant of familial adenomatous polyposis, in which intestinal adenomatous polyps are found in conjunction with osteomas of the skull or long bones, epidermoid cysts, and fibromatosis (desmoid tumors). A less common variant of familial polyposis is **Turcot syndrome,** which features medulloblastoma and glioblastoma multiforme but fewer polyps. Onset of polyps in these syndromes begins at puberty, and symptoms usually begin between 20 and 30 years of age, followed by carcinoma development that often is within 1 decade.

Dilation of the lumen of the appendix by mucinous secretions is termed an **appendiceal mucocele.** This mucocele most commonly occurs from a mucinous cystadenoma, but also can occur from epithelial hyperplasia or a mucinous cystadenocarcinoma. Extra-appendiceal extension in the form of peritoneal implants can occur, which can fill the peritoneal cavity with mucin, producing a serious condition known as **pseudomyxoma peritonei.**

Lipomas are the most common nonepithelial tumors of the colon and frequently are associated with intussusception. These tumors present as rounded submucosal masses, which often create acute angles with the colonic wall and are noticeably compressible. Less common benign tumors

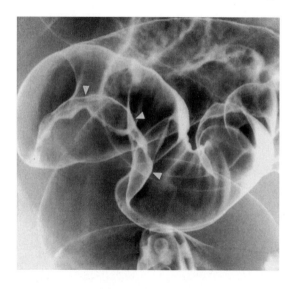

Figure 7–31. Endometrioma. Double-contrast barium enema illustrates a large mass invading the wall of the sigmoid colon and protruding into the lumen (*arrowheads*).

include leiomyomas, lymphangiomas, fibrovascular polyps, and neurofibromas. **Endometriomas** can implant on the colonic serosa (Fig. 7–31). **Leiomyomas** are common neoplasms that arise in the submucosal layer. They may ulcerate and cause bleeding.

Carcinoid tumors are potentially malignant neoplasms of the neuroendocrine system. They may arise anywhere in the colon, but most carcinoids of the large intestine originate in the rectum. Carcinoid is the most common appendiceal tumor.

Malignant Neoplasms

The **adenoma-carcinoma sequence** refers to the development of carcinoma within adenomas. This is a well-established phenomenon and is the basis for widespread screening for colon cancer, either by colonoscopy or by barium enema.

The risk for development of **adenocarcinoma** in an adenoma depends on the size of the adenoma and the degree of cellular dysplasia. Size is the most important factor, with adenomas less than 1 cm having less than 1% chance of containing a malignancy, whereas adenomas between 1 and 2 cm have 10% risk, and there is 50% risk for adenomas greater than 2 cm in diameter.

Most adenocarcinomas of the colon begin within adenomatous polyps but with growth become flat, plaquelike masses. With continued growth, the masses become either large polypoid bulky lesions or infiltrating lesions that may culminate in what is referred to as an "apple-core" lesion (Fig. 7–32).

The gastrointestinal tract is the most common site of extranodal **non-Hodgkin's lymphoma.** The colon is involved much less often than the stomach or the small bowel. Most lymphomas are seen in the cecal region, but any segment may be involved, including the rectum. The radiographic appearance of lymphoma is as varied as elsewhere in the gastrointestinal tract, including small ulcerated masses, large bulky masses, constricting lesions simulating carcinoma, and a polyposis form that simulates the familial polyposis syndromes (Fig. 7–33). Malignancy can spread to the colon via mesenteric reflections (such as the gastrocolic ligament and transverse mesocolon), direct invasion, intraperitoneal seeding, and hematogenous metastases (Fig. 7–34).

Miscellaneous Conditions

Pneumatosis coli, the presence of air in the wall of the colon, can be a benign or serious condition. Pneumatosis coli can be divided into two categories: pneumatosis cystoides coli and pneumatosis intestinalis. **Pneumatosis cystoides coli** is a mostly asymptomatic condition characterized by large round collections of air in the colonic wall. It is associated with benign causes, such as iatrogenic mucosal injury (i.e., colonoscopy, rectal tube insertion, surgery). **Pneumatosis intestinalis** is a symptomatic condition that is associated with potentially serious conditions, such as infectious colitis, necrotizing enterocolitis, bowel infarction, typhlitis, and toxic megacolon (Fig. 7–35). It

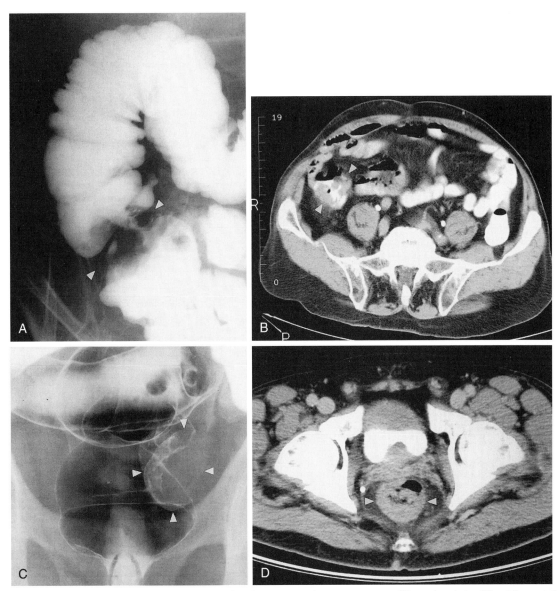

Figure 7–32. Colonic adenocarcinoma. Single-contrast barium enema **(A)** and pelvic CT with rectal contrast **(B)** reveal a classic "apple-core" appearance of an adenocarcinoma *(arrowheads)* infiltrating the cecal wall and severely and abruptly narrowing the lumen. Double-contrast barium enema **(C)** and pelvic CT **(D)** in different patients show eccentric masses invading the rectum *(arrowheads)*.

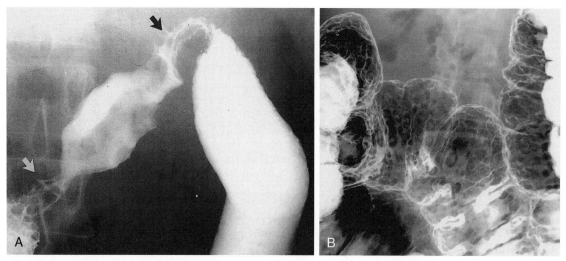

Figure 7–33. Colonic lymphoma. Barium enemas demonstrate the various appearances of colonic lymphoma: Aneurysmal dilation between strictures *(arrows)* **(A)** and the polyposis **(B)** form diffusely involving the colon, with inner dimples representing nodules containing central collections of barium.

typically features linear intramural gas collections.

Intussusception is the prolapse of one part of the bowel (intussusceptum) into the lumen of an adjoining segment (intussuscipiens). Several varieties of intussusception can be seen in the colon, the most common being ileocecal and ileocolic. In ileocecal intussusception, the ileocecal valve prolapses into the cecum, dragging the ileum along with it. In ileocolic intussusception, the ileum prolapses through the ileocecal valve into the cecum. Although about 20% of cases are idiopathic, lesions such as colonic neoplasms (especially polyps and lipomas) or a Meckel diverticulum can provide the lead point for intussusception. Diagnosis can be suggested by a localized ileus, classically in the right lower quadrant, or visualization of the intussusception mass. Confirmation can be obtained with air or contrast enema, ultrasound, or CT (Fig. 7–36). On ultrasound and CT, the intussusception mass has a characteristic "pseudo-kidney" appearance given by the invaginated mesenteric fat surrounded by bowel wall. In children, reduc-

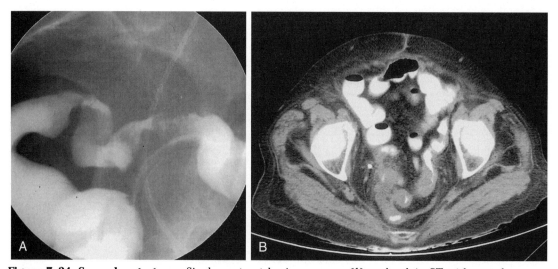

Figure 7–34. Serosal metastases. Single-contrast barium enema **(A)** and pelvic CT with rectal contrast **(B)** display multifocal narrowing of the lumen of the sigmoid colon, representing serosal metastases from cervical cancer.

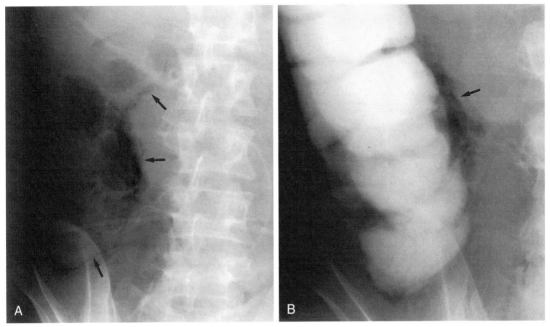

Figure 7–35. Pneumatosis intestinalis. Conventional radiograph **(A)** and subsequent single-contrast barium enema **(B)** exhibit intramural collections of air *(arrows)* that occurred as a complication of cytomegalovirus colitis.

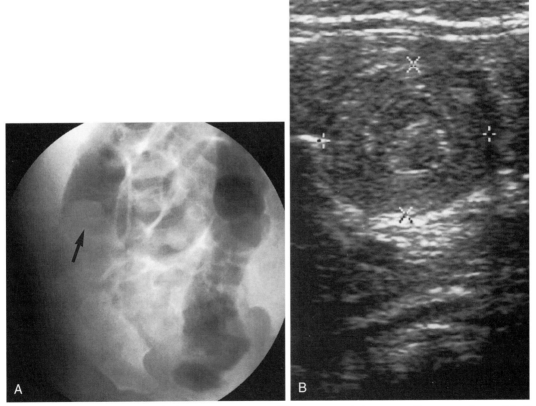

Figure 7–36. Intussusception. A, Air-contrast enema illustrates an intussusception mass *(arrow)* in the ascending colon. **B,** Ultrasound reveals the classic "pseudo-kidney" appearance of the intussusception mass (between calipers), with central echogenicity representing invaginated fat, surrounded by bowel wall. **(B,** From Williamson SL: Essentials of Pediatric Radiology. Philadelphia, WB Saunders, 2001.)

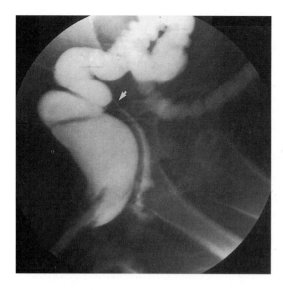

Figure 7–37. Rectovaginal fistula. Single-contrast barium enema demonstrates communication with the vagina through a fistulous tract *(arrow)*.

tion can be attempted fluoroscopically either by air or contrast enema.

Colonic fistulas can form to essentially any adjacent structure, including the biliary system, duodenum, stomach, small bowel, bladder, vagina (Fig. 7–37), and skin. Fistulas of the colon are usually the result of infection, adjacent inflammation, inflammatory bowel disease, radiation, surgery, or carcinoma.

Colitis cystica profunda is a rare condition in which mucinous cysts are found in the wall of the colon. Involvement usually is confined to the rectum and almost always occurs in adults. Symptoms include vague abdominal pain, bleeding, diarrhea, and rectal prolapse. The radiologic findings of multiple radiolucent mural-based cystic structures are similar to pneumatosis coli.

Often found in conjunction with cutaneous urticaria, **colonic urticaria** generally are associated with drug reactions. On barium enema, urticaria of the colon are seen as a mosaic of polygonal plaques, which represent focal areas of submucosal edema (Fig. 7–38).

Gastrointestinal hemorrhage can be difficult to localize and can occur from a variety of conditions, such as diverticular disease, angiodysplasia, neoplasms, trauma, ischemia, and inflammatory bowel disease. **Gastrointestinal bleeding studies** are performed most commonly with technetium 99m–labeled red blood cells. This examination is particularly useful in localizing periodically bleeding lesions because angiography can be used for localization only during active bleeding.

Most cases of **cathartic colon** were reported in the 1940s and 1950s, among women who used laxatives for 10 to 15 years. Laxatives containing podophyllin,

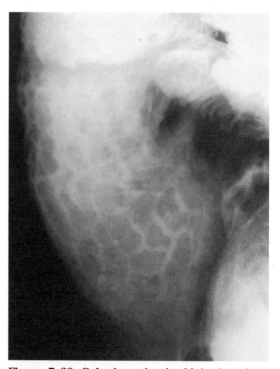

Figure 7–38. Colonic urticaria. Multiple polygonal plaques representing focal areas of submucosal edema from urticaria are seen in the cecum on a single-contrast barium enema.

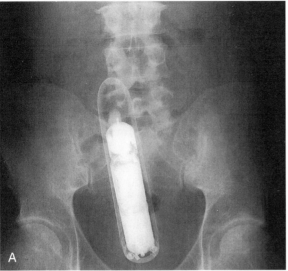

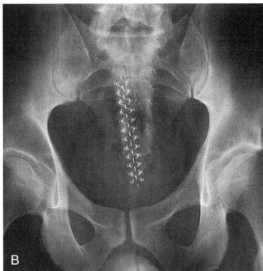

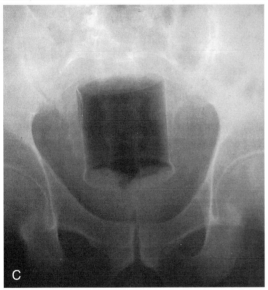

Figure 7-39. Rectal foreign bodies. Abdominal radiographs show various intentionally inserted rectal foreign bodies that became unretrievable, prompting visits to the emergency department for extraction: **A**, Vibrator containing two C-cell batteries. **B**, Hairbrush. **C**, Vienna sausage can.

which no longer is used, seem to have been the causative factor. Cathartic colon is now a radiologic curiosity and is seen rarely. Prolonged use of cathartics can induce structural changes in the colon and is manifested radiographically by absent or decreased haustra and tubular areas of narrowing. Involvement usually is proximal, but the entire colon can be affected in severe cases.

Trauma of the colon is rare and generally occurs from penetrating injury, hypoperfusion, or impalement. Other traumatic injuries can arise from intentional insertion of foreign bodies or iatrogenically from colonoscopy.

Colorectal foreign bodies are seen commonly in emergency department patients. The objects often are placed intentionally for sexual gratification purposes and become unretrievable. Prisoners and drug traffickers have been known to use this route to hide illicit objects. Reported foreign bodies include vibrators, broom handles, fruits and vegetables, bottles, flashlights, live artillery shells, and light bulbs (Fig. 7-39).

Suggested Readings

Gore RM, Levine MS, Laufer I: Textbook of Gastrointestinal Radiology, 2nd ed. Philadelphia, WB Saunders, 2000.

Houston JD, Davis M: Fundamentals of Fluoroscopy. Philadelphia, WB Saunders, 2001.

Laufer I, Levine MS, Rubesin SE: Double Contrast Gastrointestinal Radiology, 3rd ed. Philadelphia, WB Saunders, 1999.

Marshak RH, Lindner AE, Maklansky D: Radiology of the Colon. Philadelphia, WB Saunders, 1980.

EIGHT

Liver

JULIE A. LOCKEN, M.D.

Normal Anatomy

A basic knowledge of normal hepatic anatomy and vascular supply is essential in understanding the disease processes that involve the liver. The liver is unique in having a dual blood supply, with approximately 75% originating from the portal venous system and 25% arising from the hepatic artery. The hepatic veins are responsible for drainage of filtered blood from the liver into the inferior vena cava (IVC).

The liver is divided into three functional lobes: the right lobe, the left lobe, and the caudate lobe (Fig. 8–1). The **right lobe** is divided into anterior and posterior segments, whereas the **left lobe** is divided into medial and lateral segments. The **caudate lobe** is positioned posteriorly and is separated from the remainder of the liver by the fissure for the ligamentum venosum. The major hepatic veins course between the lobes and segments of the liver, helping to define the anatomy for various imaging modalities.

The anterior segment of the right lobe is separated from the medial segment of the left lobe by the **main interlobar fissure,** which contains the middle hepatic vein. The right hepatic vein separates the anterior and posterior segments of the right lobe. The left hepatic vein separates the medial and lateral segments of the left lobe. The portal veins generally course centrally through the different segments and are intrasegmental.

Imaging Modalities

Ultrasonography is often the first examination performed in patients with abnormal liver function tests, right upper quadrant pain, or suspected malignancy. Ultrasound is noninvasive and an excellent screening tool. With the advent of color Doppler imaging, hepatic vascular abnormalities can be identified readily; this is useful in the evaluation of transplant patients to determine patency of hepatic vessels, particularly the IVC, portal vein, hepatic veins, and hepatic ar-

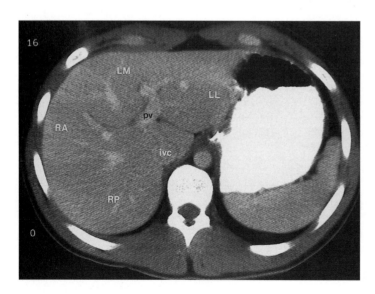

Figure 8–1. Anatomy of the liver. Contrasted CT reveals the normal anatomy of the liver: right lobe, posterior segment (RP); right lobe, anterior segment (RA); left lobe, medial segment (LM); left lobe, lateral segment (LL); main portal vein (pv); inferior vena cava (ivc). The caudate lobe is seen anterior to the inferior vena cava.

tery. In color Doppler imaging, shades of red typically refer to blood flowing toward the transducer, whereas shades of blue refer to blood flowing away from the transducer.

Multiple protocols for **computed tomography** (CT) have proved useful in evaluating diffuse and focal liver abnormalities. It is important to understand the basic rationale behind these techniques to tailor the examination for each patient. The most often employed techniques use an intravenous bolus of iodinated contrast with imaging performed in different phases of hepatic enhancement. Noncontrasted CT may be used in patients who are allergic to iodinated contrast agents, who have poor renal function, or in whom a high-density lesion is suspected.

When searching for hypervascular lesions, such as hepatoma or metastatic disease, a three-phase technique often is employed. Initially, noncontrasted images of the liver are obtained. Then an intravenous bolus of 100 to 150 mL of iodinated contrast is administered, and imaging is performed in the hepatic arterial and portal venous phases of enhancement. The rationale behind this technique is that primary and secondary malignancies of the liver typically have hepatic arterial supply, whereas benign entities and normal liver parenchyma have primarily portal venous supply.

Magnetic resonance imaging (MRI) is used to a lesser extent than either ultrasound or CT, in part because of availability and cost. Despite these limitations, MRI can be an adjunctive method of evaluation in patients who are allergic to iodinated contrast agents, who have poor renal function, or in whom the CT findings are equivocal. Although a variety of sequences have been employed, most of which are beyond the scope of this chapter, the basic spin echo T1-weighted and T2-weighted sequences are often sufficient. Spoiled gradient echo breath-hold sequences are employed for evaluating hepatic disease because intravenous contrast (gadolinium DTPA) can be used more efficiently. Fat typically is of hyperintense signal (bright) on a T1-weighted image. Water or edema is usually of hyperintense signal on a T2-weighted image. MRI often can be helpful in the characterization of a small (<2 cm) benign hemangioma that is equivocal on CT examination.

Nuclear medicine imaging is not often employed to evaluate liver disease. It is indicated, however, in certain situations. As mentioned previously, evaluation of hemangiomas can be fraught with difficulties. Technetium 99m–labeled red blood cell single-photon emission computed tomography (SPECT) can be helpful in the evaluation of lesions larger than 2 cm. Sulfur colloid liver-spleen imaging sometimes is useful in patients with cirrhosis and suspected portal hypertension. Focal areas of decreased activity in the liver on liver-spleen scanning is a nonspecific finding, and the differential diagnosis is extensive. Gallium scans seldom are used but can be helpful in some cases, showing abnormal increased activity in primary hepatomas, metastases, abscesses, and lymphoma.

Structural Abnormalities

After hemangiomas, the second most common benign hepatic lesion is the **simple cyst,** which may be solitary or multiple (Fig. 8–2). Occurring in approximately 2% to 10% of the population, cysts usually are asymptomatic, are of unknown cause, and are seen with increasing frequency with age. Cysts are variable in size and are lined with cuboidal epithelium. They are more common in women aged 50 to 70 years. Cysts are associated with other disease processes, such as tuberous sclerosis and polycystic kidney disease. Approximately 40% of patients with polycystic kidney disease also have cysts in the liver, and 60% of patients with multiple cysts in the liver have polycystic kidney disease.

The sonographic criteria necessary for diagnosis of simple cysts require that the cysts are anechoic, have posterior acoustic enhancement, and are well defined or have imperceptible walls. The accuracy of ultrasound for diagnosis of simple cysts is 95% to 99%. Only rarely does a cystic metastasis mimic a benign simple cyst. The typical appearance of a simple cyst on CT is a sharply demarcated water-density lesion with no perceptible wall and no contrast enhancement. MRI usually reveals homogeneous low intensity on T1-weighted images and homogeneous high intensity on T2-weighted images.

Focal nodular hyperplasia is a nonencapsulated nodular mass that is more common in women and usually is asymptomatic. It is believed to be a vascular or hamartomatous

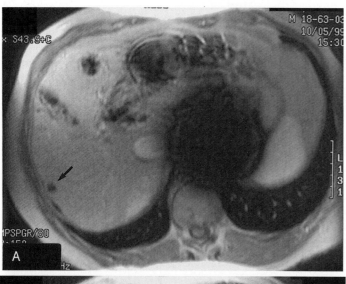

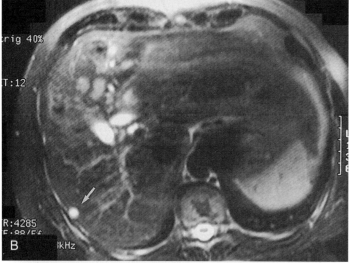

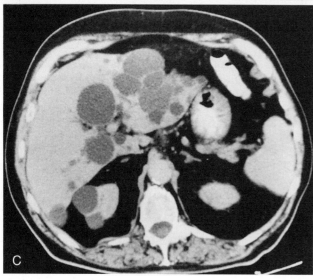

Figure 8–2. Simple cyst. Appearances of simple hepatic cysts on various imaging modalities: A small round low signal lesion *(arrow)* on T1-weighted MRI **(A)** that has high T2 signal *(arrow)* on T2-weighted MRI **(B);** and multiple low-attenuation, nonenhancing lesions on contrasted CT **(C)** in a patient with polycystic kidney disease.

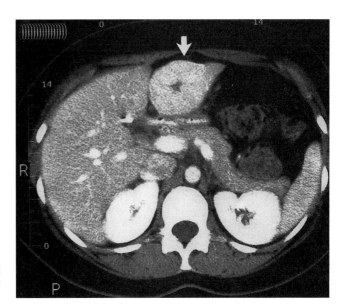

Figure 8–3. Focal nodular hyperplasia. Contrasted CT exhibits an enhancing mass *(arrow)* with a central scar in the left lobe of the liver.

malformation and is composed of normal hepatocytes, Kupffer cells, and bile ducts with abnormal arrangement. The lesions are usually less than 5 cm in diameter and most commonly are found peripherally in the right lobe. The classic appearance is a solitary, well-circumscribed mass with a central stellate scar of fibrosis. The central scar is seen in only 20% of cases, however.

The lesion is of variable echogenicity on ultrasound, and typically the central scar, if present, does not enhance with iodinated contrast on CT (Fig. 8–3). The major diagnostic consideration is fibrolamellar carcinoma, which also can contain a central hypodense area. MRI may be of help in discerning these two possibilities. Both lesions typically are hypointense or isointense on T1-weighted images. On T2-weighted images, the central scar is hyperintense in focal nodular hyperplasia, whereas it is hypointense in fibrolamellar carcinoma. Nuclear medicine sulfur colloid scans are normal in approximately 50%, have a focal photopenic defect in 40%, and have a focal area of increased activity in 10%. Angiography classically shows a "spoke-wheel" pattern of increased vascularity.

Focal fatty infiltration is more common in the left lobe of the liver and is associated with obesity, alcohol abuse, steroids, and hyperalimentation. Bandlike geographic areas of increased echogenicity in a lobar or segmental distribution generally are seen on ultrasound. Focal fatty infiltrate does not exhibit mass effect on adjacent vessels. Patchy areas of decreased attenuation are seen on CT (Fig. 8–4).

Hepatic Infections

Common causes of **hepatic abscesses** are bacterial, parasitic, and fungal. Approximately 85% to 90% of abscesses are bacterial in origin. Bacteria usually gain access to the liver via the biliary system or portal vein. The two most common bacteria to infect

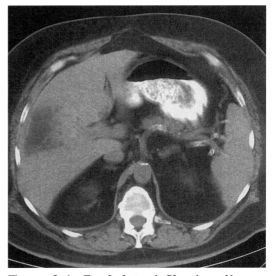

Figure 8–4. Focal fatty infiltration. Noncontrasted CT illustrates a focal area of decreased attenuation in the right lobe of the liver, representing an area of fatty infiltration.

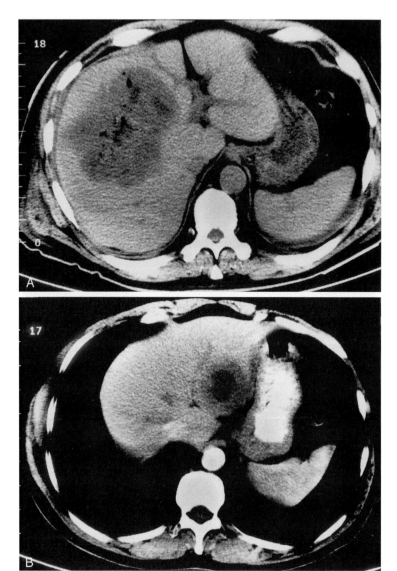

Figure 8–5. Pyogenic liver abscesses. CT scans in two patients display a large air-containing pyogenic abscess in the right lobe of the liver **(A)** and a smaller abscess in the left lobe that does not contain air **(B).**

the liver are *Escherichia coli* and anaerobes. Possible causes include iatrogenic, underlying biliary disease, diverticulitis, trauma, and inflammatory bowel disease, as well as other less common entities. Patients present with typical signs of infection, including fever, pain, diarrhea, leukocytosis, and elevated liver function tests. Most abscesses occur in the right lobe, and there is a near 100% mortality if left untreated. With treatment, which usually consists of percutaneous or surgical drainage and antibiotics, there is 10% to 15% mortality.

Sonographically, abscesses usually are heterogeneous, rounded masses with irregular thickened walls and poor peripheral definition. Internal echoes with possible

fluid-fluid levels and debris are common. Acoustic shadowing is indicative of a gas-containing lesion. CT shows a heterogeneous lesion with irregular margins with possible peripheral enhancement (Fig. 8–5). Internal septations or papillary projections are common. Approximately 20% of these lesions contain gas. Diagnosis is usually fairly certain when combined with clinical suspicion; however, cystic or necrotic metastatic disease (e.g., ovarian neoplasms or leiomyosarcoma) sometimes can be a differential diagnostic consideration. Nuclear medicine studies show a cold defect on sulfur colloid imaging and increased activity with gallium imaging. Hepatocellular carcinoma and metastatic disease can have a similar appearance on nuclear medicine studies.

In North America, only about 10% of abscesses involving the liver are of parasitic origin. Parasitic causes are much more common in third world countries. The two most common infections are due to either *Entamoeba histolytica* (amebiasis) or *Echinococcus granulososis* (hydatid cyst disease).

Amebiasis is a primary infection of the colon that is transmitted by the fecal-oral route. Cysts colonize the colon and gain access to the liver via the portal venous system. The sonographic and CT appearance is virtually indistinguishable from pyogenic abscesses (Fig. 8–6). They often are peripheral and classically contain "anchovy paste"–type material when aspirated. Treatment is usually pharmacologic, although abscesses can be drained percutaneously if necessary. Efficacy of therapy can be followed with ultrasound, although it may take several months for complete resolution.

Echinococcal disease presents with similar symptoms as other infections, but the clinical demographics often offer a suspected diagnosis. These abscesses are more common in the right lobe, may involve the chest, and may be multiple. They typically grow slowly and are more cystlike in appearance. Sonographically the classic descriptive terms used include "double-line" sign, "water lily" sign, and "racemose," which are used to describe the appearance of the cyst walls. There is usually a double-layered cyst with an inner germinal membrane that is the origin of *daughter cysts.* There is typically a thin calcified curvilinear wall that is depicted easily on CT and often on conventional radiographs (Fig. 8–7). There is controversy over percutaneous and surgical drainage with the possibility of anaphylactic shock.

With immunocompromised patients, there is increasing frequency of **fungal microabscesses** affecting the liver and the spleen. These microabscesses most commonly are due to opportunistic infections, such as *Candida* and other fungi (Fig. 8–8). Other organisms seen in immunosuppressed patients include *Pneumocystis carinii* (multiple hyperechoic foci), cytomegalovirus (multiple focal echogenic lesions), and mycobacteria. Attempts at biopsy to obtain tissue diagnosis often are unrewarding. Two neoplastic processes affecting the liver in immunocompromised patients are Kaposi sarcoma (periportal low densities) and lymphoma (variable appearance).

Diffuse Hepatic Disease

Fatty infiltration of the liver is a reversible process that is caused by triglyceride accumulation within hepatocytes. Fatty infiltration is common and can be caused by a variety of disorders, including alcoholism, diabetes mellitus, obesity, total parenteral hyperalimentation, exogenous steroids, malnutrition, glycogen storage disease, and chemotherapeutic agents. Removal or correc-

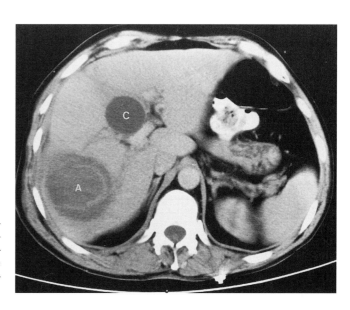

Figure 8–6. Amebic abscess. Contrasted CT indicates a peripherally enhancing amebic abscess (A) in the posterior segment of the right lobe of the liver. A simple cyst (C) is just anterolateral to the main portal vein.

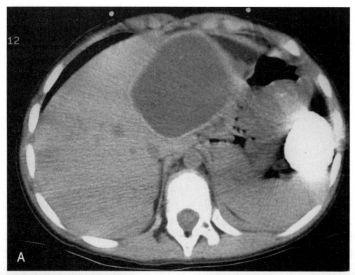

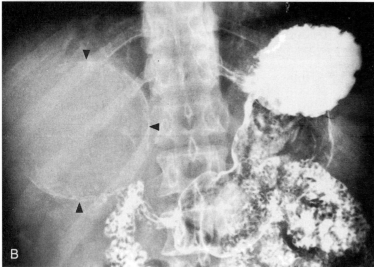

Figure 8–7. Echinococcal cyst. A, Noncontrasted CT reveals a large, peripherally calcified echinococcal cyst in a 5-year-old girl. **B,** Upper gastrointestinal series in another patient incidentally exhibits a rim of calcification *(arrowheads)* from an hepatic echinococcal cyst.

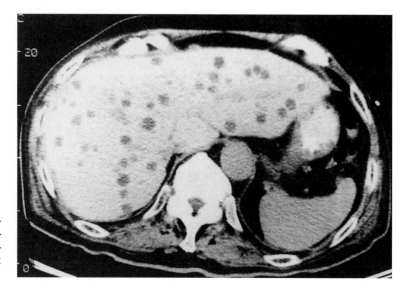

Figure 8–8. Fungal microabscesses. Contrasted CT demonstrates multiple low-attenuation lesions that represent fungal microabscesses.

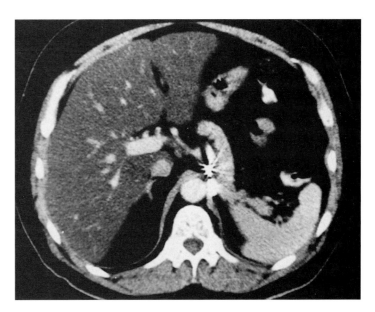

Figure 8–9. Fatty infiltration. Noncontrasted CT illustrates a diffusely low-attenuation liver from fatty infiltration.

tion of the underlying abnormality typically reverses the process.

The typical sonographic appearance of fatty infiltration is increased liver echogenicity, which may be focal or diffuse. It sometimes is helpful to compare the echogenicity of liver to surrounding organs, such as the kidney, in evaluation for possible fatty deposition. On noncontrasted CT, the fatty deposits cause decreased attenuation of hepatic parenchyma. After administration of intravenous contrast, the hepatic and portal veins are seen easily as a result of the surrounding low attenuation of parenchyma (Fig. 8–9).

In addition to focal fatty infiltration, there can be areas of **focal fatty sparing.** These areas can create the appearance of pseudomasses and always should be considered if there is a question of a mass seen in a liver with fat deposition. Characteristic locations for sparing include the periportal regions, caudate lobe, and adjacent to the gallbladder fossa.

Deposition of iron in the liver may be primary or secondary. **Primary hemochromatosis** is an autosomal recessive metabolic abnormality that causes iron to be deposited in hepatocytes, pancreas, and the myocardium. These patients have increased incidence of hepatocellular carcinoma. **Secondary hemochromatosis** results in deposition of iron in the reticuloendothelial cells of the liver and the spleen that is caused by multiple blood transfusions.

Generally, on ultrasound the echogenicity of the liver is normal in hemochromatosis.

CT shows diffuse increased attenuation of liver parenchyma (Fig. 8–10). MRI shows decreased signal on T1-weighted and T2-weighted images, but it is most significant on the T2-weighted images when compared with the signal intensities of normal liver. MRI can be useful if other imaging modalities are equivocal.

Although there are numerous causes of **cirrhosis,** the most common cause in North America is alcohol abuse. Pathologically, cirrhosis consists of different amounts of hepatocyte necrosis, fibrosis, fatty infiltration, and nodular regeneration, which may be macronodular or micronodular in appearance. Alcohol tends to cause the macronodular form, whereas chronic viral hepatitis is a more likely cause of the micronodular form. Regardless of cause, several characteristic findings are evident on imaging studies.

The ultrasound appearance of advanced cirrhosis typically reveals a contracted liver with relative enlargement of the lateral segment of the left lobe and caudate. Associated findings are a coarse echotexture of the liver parenchyma, presumably secondary to fatty infiltration and fibrosis, and a nodular irregular liver surface, which often is seen well secondary to concomitant ascites. Noncontrasted CT may show either heterogeneous or homogeneous decreased attenuation of the hepatic parenchyma, depending on amounts of fatty infiltration, fibrosis, and regenerating nodules. After intravenous contrast administration, areas of fibrosis and regeneration may become isoattenuating

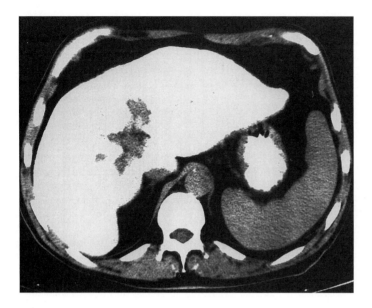

Figure 8–10. Hemochromatosis. Noncontrasted CT displays a diffusely high-attenuation liver that differs markedly in attenuation from the spleen in a patient with hemochromatosis.

with parenchyma. MRI may be essentially normal with slightly heterogeneous signal intensity on T1-weighted and T2-weighted imaging. Areas of hepatic fibrosis may be of low signal on T1-weighted images, whereas these areas may be of high signal on T2-weighted images.

In patients with cirrhosis, associated findings of **portal venous hypertension** are seen on many types of imaging studies. Ultrasound, CT, and MRI may show ascites, splenomegaly, and portosystemic varices (Fig. 8–11). The most commonly identified varices by ultrasound and CT are the paraumbilical vein, which runs in the falciform ligament,

and splenorenal or gastrorenal veins. Doppler ultrasound can determine if flow is hepatofugal (away from the liver) or hepatopedal (toward the liver).

Acute hepatitis of any origin causes the hepatocytes to become edematous. Imaging modalities show nonspecific findings, and clinical correlation is important. Ultrasound may be entirely normal in acute hepatitis or may show the classic finding of decreased echogenicity of the parenchyma with prominence of the portal venous system, causing a "starry sky" appearance. **Chronic hepatitis** typically shows no definite abnormalities on ultrasound, but there may be a coarsely

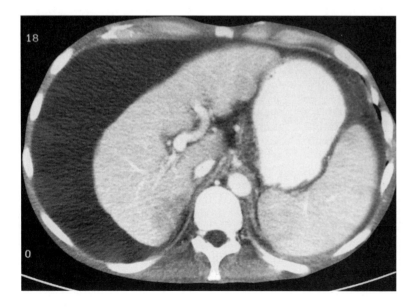

Figure 8–11. Cirrhosis. Contrasted CT illustrates splenomegaly and a small contracted liver that is displaced centrally by ascitic fluid.

echogenic parenchymal pattern. CT and MRI typically are not used in evaluating acute hepatitis.

Benign Neoplasms

Hepatic adenomas are most common in women of childbearing age and are linked to oral contraceptives, anabolic steroids, and glycogen storage diseases. Hepatic adenomas are composed of slightly atypical hepatocytes with an increased amount of glycogen and fat. They do not contain bile ducts or central portal veins and have absent or decreased Kupffer cells with abnormal function. Hepatic adenomas usually are asymptomatic but can present with pain if they become hemorrhagic and necrotic because they are hypervascular lesions. Adenomas are considered to be a clinically significant lesion because of the propensity for hemorrhage.

Sonographically, adenomas typically are well-defined circular lesions of variable echogenicity and are virtually indistinguishable from focal nodular hyperplasia. On CT, they are discrete, rounded masses of low attenuation that typically exhibit variable enhancement after iodinated contrast administration. Adenomas may have areas of increased attenuation owing to hemorrhage or decreased attenuation owing to necrosis (Fig. 8–12). On MRI, adenomas are inhomogeneous on all pulse sequences with some increased signal on T1-weighted images as a result of increased amounts of glycogen and fat. Nuclear medicine imaging shows a focal photopenic lesion with sulfur colloid scans in 80% of cases, with approximately 20% being of normal activity when compared with the remainder of the liver. There is no increased activity on gallium imaging, as is seen with hepatic abscess, hepatocellular carcinoma, and metastatic disease.

The **cavernous hemangioma** is the most common benign hepatic lesion and may be either single or multiple. It is the second most common hepatic lesion overall, with metastatic disease ranking first in frequency. Cavernous hemangiomas are present in 4% to 20% of the general population and are more common in women, increasing in incidence with age. Cavernous hemangiomas usually are asymptomatic, but rarely may hemorrhage, thrombose, or cause abdominal discomfort if large enough to exhibit mass effect. They may enlarge slowly and degenerate, calcify, or fibrose.

The most common location for a hemangioma is in the posterior segment of the right lobe, with a subcapsular or peripheral predominance. The usual sonographic appearance of a hemangioma is a well-circumscribed, round or oval, homogeneous hyperechoic lesion. The larger the size of the lesion, the more likely it will be more heterogeneous with areas of degeneration. Doppler imaging reveals no evidence of increased flow because the hemangioma is composed of vascular channels lined with endothelial cells that have slow flow.

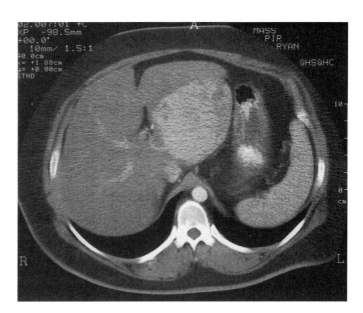

Figure 8–12. Hepatic adenoma. Contrasted CT of an hepatic adenoma in a patient on oral contraceptives exhibits a large hemorrhagic and necrotic adenoma in the left lobe of the liver.

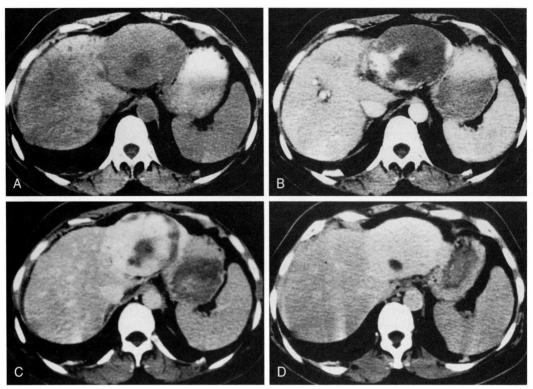

Figure 8–13. Hemangioma. CTs of an hemangioma of the left lobe of the liver in various phases of imaging: **A,** Noncontrasted. **B,** Arterial phase of enhancement (30 seconds). **C,** Portal venous phase of enhancement (60 seconds). **D,** Delayed enhancement (3 minutes). The mass is observed to fill in gradually from the periphery after intravenous contrast administration.

On noncontrasted CT, the appearance is usually that of a well-circumscribed, low-density ovoid lesion, but it can be of mixed densities. The classic appearance after an intravenous bolus of iodinated contrast is initial peripheral nodular enhancement with complete filling on delayed images (Fig. 8–13). CT technique consists of a rapid bolus with dynamic, serial imaging at a single level to document progression of enhancement from peripheral to central during 0 to 10 minutes. One of the difficulties with this technique is that necrotic metastatic disease may have a similar response, and larger hemangiomas may show atypical enhancement.

Additional studies, such as MRI or nuclear medicine SPECT imaging, may be helpful. SPECT imaging with technetium 99m–tagged red blood cells is most beneficial if the suspected lesion is greater than 2 cm in size. The hemangioma shows decreased activity on early images with increased activity on delayed images. MRI can be useful if the lesion is less than 2 cm. The typical MRI appearance is a well-defined, homogeneous mass with hypointense or isointense signal on T1-weighted images and marked hyperintense signal on T2-weighted images. Additionally, after a bolus of gadolinium, there is peripheral to central enhancement, which is similar to that described for CT. There are some difficulties with this procedure as well, however. Metastatic lesions may exhibit a similar enhancement pattern, but they usually enhance sooner and have quicker washout on delayed imaging.

Malignant Neoplasms

The most common primary visceral malignancy worldwide is **hepatocellular carcinoma** (hepatoma). In industrialized countries, the most common predisposing condition is alcoholic cirrhosis, whereas in third world countries, the most common cause is chronic hepatitis. Additional predisposing conditions include Wilson disease, hemochromatosis, and glycogen storage diseases. Hepatocellular carcinoma occurs much more commonly in men with approximately a 6:1 ratio and is most frequent between ages 60 and 70.

Pathologically, there are three histologic patterns: solitary, multiple nodular, and diffuse infiltrative. Venous extension is common, with the portal vein more often involved than the hepatic veins (30% to 60% versus 15%). Vascular invasion can occur early and does not indicate inoperability. Associated clinical findings include increased alpha-fetoprotein levels in greater than 70%, increased liver function tests, weight loss, right upper quadrant pain, ascites, and hepatomegaly. The prognosis is generally poor, with greater than 90% mortality within 5 years. The average survival is approximately 6 months.

The ultrasound appearance of hepatocellular carcinoma can be quite variable, ranging from a discrete hypoechoic mass to diffusely infiltrative that is essentially undetectable by sonographic methods. Hepatomas are extremely difficult to detect in a severely cirrhotic liver with coarse echotexture, and as a screening tool, ultrasound is relatively insensitive. On noncontrasted CT, a hepatoma is typically a hypodense mass, but sometimes can have areas of increased attenuation (Fig. 8–14). Approximately 80% show some enhancement that occurs in the hepatic arterial phase. MRI shows hyperintense or isointense signal intensity on T1-weighted images with hyperintensity on T2-weighted images in most cases. Nuclear medicine studies exhibit a focal photopenic defect on sulfur colloid scans with an area of increased activity on gallium imaging. Angiography rarely is done, but typically shows neovascularity, arteriovenous shunting, and a dilated hepatic artery.

Fibrolamellar carcinoma is a histologic subtype of hepatocellular carcinoma that typically occurs in younger individuals without predisposing cirrhosis and has a better prognosis. Fibrolamellar carcinoma more often is resectable and usually does not have an elevated alpha-fetoprotein level. It tends to be a solitary mass of variable echogenicity on ultrasound. The classic CT appearance is a well-defined mass with a central area of low density, similar to the stellate scar described in focal nodular hyperplasia. MRI can be helpful to differentiate the two because the central scar is of decreased signal intensity on T1-weighted and T2-weighted images in fibrolamellar carcinoma.

Metastases are the most common hepatic malignancy. The typical primary tumor is often of gastrointestinal origin (colon or stomach), but lung, breast, and pancreas also are common sources. Dissemination to the liver occurs through the portal vein, lymphatics, or hepatic artery. Patients may present with hepatomegaly or abnormal liver function tests. Lesions typically are multiple and involve both lobes of the liver.

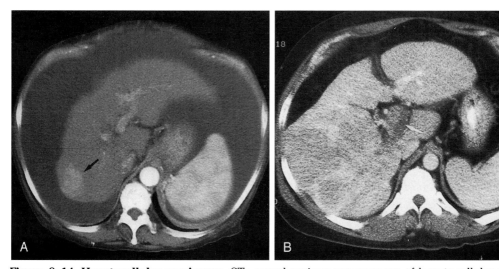

Figure 8–14. Hepatocellular carcinoma. CTs reveal various appearances of hepatocellular carcinoma: **A,** Arterial phase enhancement of a small mass in the posterior segment of the right lobe of the liver *(arrow).* **B,** Large, heterogeneously enhancing mass occupying the right lobe, with a large thrombus in the portal vein *(arrow).*

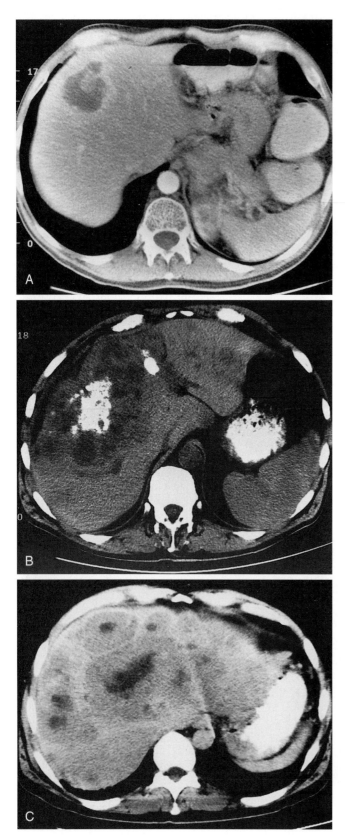

Figure 8–15. Hepatic metastases. Various CT appearances of hepatic metastases: **A,** Peripheral enhancement of a metastatic renal cell carcinoma in the anterior segment of the right lobe of the liver. **B,** Calcification of a large metastasis of a mucinous adenocarcinoma of the colon. **C,** Multiple necrotic carcinoid metastases distributed throughout the liver.

Metastases are more often calcified than are primary liver tumors.

Multiple appearances for metastatic disease have been described, including discrete hypoechoic, discrete hyperechoic, target, calcified, cystic, and diffusely inhomogeneous (Fig. 8–15). Echogenic metastases tend to be of gastrointestinal origin, but also can be seen in carcinoid tumors, renal cell carcinomas, choriocarcinomas, and islet cell tumors. Calcified metastases tend to be from mucinous colon carcinoma, although they also can be seen in ovarian cystadenocarcinoma, neuroblastoma, leiomyosarcoma, and osteogenic sarcoma. Lymphoma often is hypoechoic and can be diffusely infiltrative. Breast and lung metastases can be diffusely infiltrative. CT shows a variable presentation. An important differentiating factor from benign lesions is that metastatic disease as well as primary liver tumors typically show some degree of enhancement in the hepatic arterial phase, whereas benign lesions usually exhibit contrast enhancement in the portal venous phase of enhancement.

Miscellaneous Conditions

Portal vein thrombosis occurs in association with several hepatic disease processes. Common causes of thrombosis of the portal venous system include pancreatitis, cirrhosis, hepatocellular carcinoma, and ascending cholangitis. Less common causes include hypercoagulable states and trauma. Thrombosis can involve any or all portions of the portal venous system.

Imaging studies best used to diagnose portal venous thrombosis include ultrasound, CT, and MRI. Ultrasound typically shows an echogenic focus within a portal vein. Contrasted CT shows lack of normal enhancement of a portal vein, possibly with a low-density clot seen within the lumen of the portal vein, or, alternatively, if the vein is totally occluded, multiple periportal collateral vessels may be present. Contrasted MRI findings include lack of enhancement of the portal vein, with an intraluminal low signal thrombus (Fig. 8–16A). Additionally, indirect CT and MRI findings of portal vein thrombosis may include an entity called **transient hepatic attenuation differences.** This phenomenon is related to alterations in hepatic blood supply, with the hepatic artery now supplying the segment of liver previously supplied by the thrombosed portal vein; this causes a transient segment of hyperattenuating liver during the late arterial phase on CT and MRI (Fig. 8–16B).

Budd-Chiari syndrome is caused by obstruction of hepatic venous outflow, which may be either intrahepatic or extrahepatic. Although there are numerous causes of Budd-Chiari syndrome, the most often en-

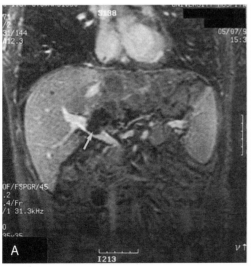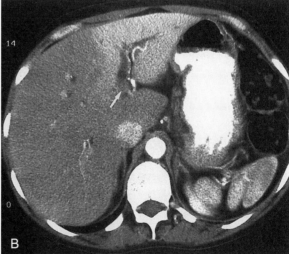

Figure 8–16. Portal vein thrombosis. A, Coronal gadolinium-enhanced magnetic resonance venogram shows heterogeneity of the left lobe of the liver as well as a large, low-intensity thrombus *(arrow)* extending into the lumen of the main portal vein. **B,** Contrasted CT reveals a left portal vein thrombus *(arrow)* and associated transient hepatic attenuation differences.

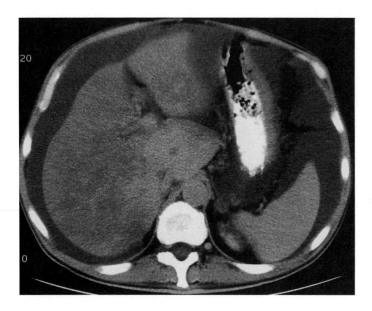

Figure 8–17. Budd-Chiari syndrome. Noncontrasted CT displays a mottled appearance of the liver, with sparing of the caudate lobe and associated surrounding ascitic fluid.

countered is idiopathic. Additional causes include tumor thrombus, trauma, pregnancy, hypercoagulable states, sepsis, dehydration, and certain drugs. Budd-Chiari syndrome is more common in women, and patients often present with acute onset of abdominal pain.

The initial imaging modality usually is ultrasound with Doppler evaluation of flow in the hepatic veins and IVC. Possible findings include actual thrombus in hepatic veins or IVC, difficulty in visualizing hepatic veins, thick echogenic venous walls, or collateral vessels. In chronic Budd-Chiari syndrome, there often is ascites and enlargement of the caudate lobe. These two findings also are

seen on CT (Fig. 8–17). There is often patchy inhomogeneous enhancement of liver parenchyma with a tendency for early central enhancement and subsequent washout, followed by delayed peripheral enhancement. MRI typically shows either absent flow or narrowing of hepatic veins or IVC. It is important to look for associated findings of ascites and an enlarged caudate lobe.

Passive hepatic congestion most often is caused by congestive heart failure. There is decreased hepatic blood flow related to increased central venous pressure, leading to hepatic venous hypertension. Clinically, patients typically have hepatomegaly, upper

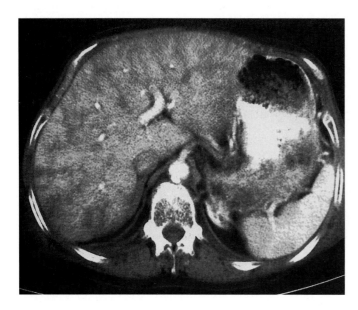

Figure 8–18. Passive hepatic congestion. Contrasted CT exhibits mottled hepatic enhancement in a patient with venous congestion from congestive heart failure.

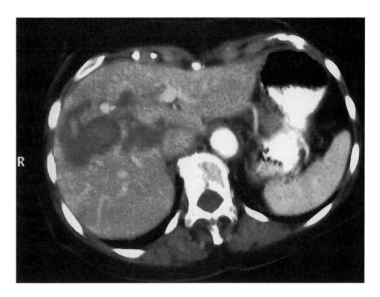

Figure 8–19. Hepatic laceration. Contrasted CT indicates a linear low-attenuation laceration of the anterior segment of the right lobe of the liver after a motor vehicle accident.

abdominal pain, and possibly elevated liver function studies.

CT and MRI findings are similar and include heterogeneous liver enhancement and enlarged hepatic veins and IVC, with possible pleural effusions, cardiomegaly, and ascites (Fig. 8–18). The key to the radiographic diagnosis is in differentiating this entity from Budd-Chiari syndrome. With passive hepatic congestion, the hepatic veins and IVC are prominent, whereas in Budd-Chiari syndrome, the hepatic veins and IVC are diminutive.

Following blunt abdominal **trauma,** the liver is the second most commonly injured organ (after the spleen). The posterior segment of the right hepatic lobe is injured most often, which is thought to be related to the relative fixation by coronary ligaments.

Contrasted CT is the method of choice for the evaluation of liver injury. **Hepatic lacerations** appear as areas of low attenuation relative to the remainder of normal enhancing liver tissue (Fig. 8–19). Lacerations most often are linear or branching, although they can be rounded. Lacerations are graded (I through IV) based on depth, location within the liver, and proximity to adjacent hepatic veins and portal veins. There typically is associated hemoperitoneum. Iso-lated **subcapsular hematomas** can occur, although they are uncommon in the setting of blunt trauma. Subcapsular hematomas are associated more often with penetrating trauma or recent percutanous biopsy. **Periportal edema** or lymphedema often is present and can be related to the liver injury itself, although it more often is thought to be related to vigorous intravenous fluid resuscitation. Lacerations tend to show healing on serial CT examinations during a 2- to 4-week period.

Suggested Readings

Friedman AC, Dachman AH: Radiology of the Liver, Biliary Tract, Pancreas, and Spleen, 2nd ed. St. Louis, Mosby-Year Book, 1994.

Haaga JR, Lanzieri CF, Sartoris DJ, Zerhouni EA: Computed Tomography and Magnetic Resonance of the Whole Body, 3rd ed. St. Louis, Mosby-Year Book, 1994.

Lee JK, Sagel SS, Stanley RJ, Heiken JP: Computed Body Tomography with MRI Correlation, 3rd ed. Philadelphia, Lippincott-Raven, 1998.

Mittelstaedt CA: General Ultrasound. New York, Churchill Livingstone, 1992.

Moss AA, Gamsu G, Genant HK: Computed Tomography of the Body with Magnetic Resonance Imaging, 2nd ed. Philadelphia, WB Saunders, 1992.

Webb WR, Brant WE, Helms CA: Fundamentals of Body CT, 2nd ed. Philadelphia, WB Saunders, 1991.

NINE

Biliary System

Danica C. Holt, M.D.

Normal Anatomy

The biliary system includes the gallbladder as well as the intrahepatic and extrahepatic bile ducts (Fig. 9–1). The **gallbladder** is a pear-shaped organ that lies inferior to the liver in a shallow fossa. Peritoneum covers the inferior and posterior surfaces, although the gallbladder may be invested completely in peritoneum and have a mesentery. The gallbladder can be divided into three parts: the **fundus, body,** and **neck.** The neck is directed toward the porta hepatis and becomes continuous with the cystic duct. The gallbladder measures approximately 10 cm in length and 3 to 5 cm in diameter when distended and can hold approximately 50 mL of bile. The gallbladder stores and concentrates the bile secreted by the liver.

The **cystic duct** is approximately 2 to 4 cm in length. The initial segment is tortuous with mucosal folds, known as **spiral valves** (of Heister), which maintain cystic duct patency. The cystic duct usually joins the **common hepatic duct** to form the common bile duct, although multiple variations are possible, as is true for the entire ductal system. The **common bile duct** is approximately 8 to 10 cm in length and 5 to 6 mm in diameter. It descends with the hepatic artery and portal vein posterior to the duodenum and pancreatic head. The duct then joins the main pancreatic duct and forms the **ampulla of Vater** before entering the duodenum of the **major papilla.** The distal common bile duct is encircled by a muscular sheath (the choledochal sphincter) before the duct's entrance to the duodenum. When this sphincter contracts, bile is forced back into the gallbladder for storage. The **sphincter of Oddi** encircles the ampulla of Vater and controls the release of bile into the duodenum.

Imaging Modalities

Multiple imaging modalities are used to study the gallbladder and biliary ductal sys-

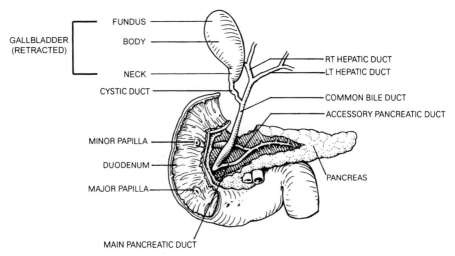

Figure 9–1. Anatomy of the biliary system. The anatomic relationship of the gallbladder, bile ducts, and pancreas to adjacent structures.

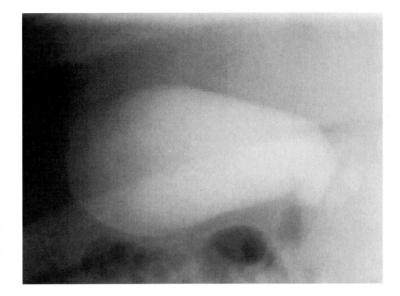

Figure 9–2. Oral cholecystogram. Radiograph of the right upper quadrant in the Trendelenburg position shows opacification of the gallbladder from oral ingestion of iopanoic acid.

tem. **Conventional radiographs** can identify some gallstones (10% to 15% are calcified), air within the biliary system, an enlarged gallbladder, small bowel ileus from cholecystitis, and a calcified gallbladder.

Oral cholecystography has been replaced by sonography as the standard for gallbladder imaging but remains useful in detecting gallstones when sonography is equivocal and is sensitive in the detection of other benign gallbladder diseases, including polypoid masses. An orally ingested iodine compound is absorbed by the intestinal mucosa, transported to the liver for conjugation, excreted into the bile, and concentrated in the gallbladder. Radiographs can be obtained fluoroscopically in various positions (Fig. 9–2).

Ultrasonography is the most widely used study to image the gallbladder, and it does not rely on gallbladder or hepatic function, in contrast to the oral cholecystogram. After 6 hours of fasting, sonography of the gallbladder is performed in the supine and decubitus positions. Normal and dilated biliary ducts are identified readily and can be measured (Fig. 9–3).

Computed tomography (CT) can detect some gallstones and dilated biliary ducts, but it is less sensitive than sonography. **Magnetic resonance imaging** (MRI) has increasing utility in noninvasive imaging of the biliary system, particularly with the proliferation of magnetic resonance cholangiopancreatography (Fig. 9–4).

Nuclear medicine imaging uses techne-

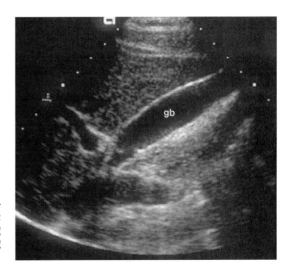

Figure 9–3. Ultrasound of the gallbladder. Transabdominal ultrasound affords optimal radiologic visualization of the gallbladder (gb) in a fasting patient. Note the thin echogenic wall surrounding anechoic bile in the lumen.

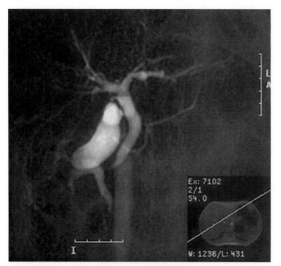

Figure 9–4. Magnetic resonance cholangiopancreatogram. Thick-slab, oblique coronal, single-shot T2 fast spin echo MRI of the abdomen allows visualization of the biliary system. The common bile duct is particularly well seen because it is dilated slightly from ampullary stenosis. The fluid in the right renal collecting system and thecal sac can be seen faintly overlying the image.

tium 99m–iminodiacetic acid (^{99m}Tc-IDA), which is injected intravenously. This compound is taken up by hepatocytes and excreted in the bile. Sequential images in the normal patient show homogeneous uptake in the liver with biliary excretion within 30 minutes (Fig. 9–5). If the gallbladder is not visualized in 1 hour, an injection of a cholecystokinin analog or ingestion of a fatty meal increases tone at the sphincter of Oddi and diverts bile to the gallbladder. Delayed images at 4 hours postinjection may be obtained. If the gallbladder still is not visualized, the cystic duct is considered obstructed. Hepatobiliary scanning is useful in other biliary diseases and is discussed under those disease categories.

Endoscopic retrograde cholangiopancreatography (ERCP) is performed by passing an endoscope into the duodenum. After cannulation of the pancreatic duct and common bile duct, iodinated contrast is injected. ERCP is advantageous when evaluating a suspected primary pancreatic carcinoma, pancreatitis and its complications, or biliary disorders. Sphincterotomy, brush biopsies, stone extraction, and biliary stent placement all can be performed through the endoscope. Similar images can be obtained with an **intraoperative cholangiogram,** in which

the cystic duct is injected with iodinated contrast (Fig. 9–6), or a **T-tube cholangiogram,** in which contrast is injected through a surgically placed T-tube. **Percutaneous transhepatic cholangiography** (PTC) is performed by interventional radiologists by successively passing a long needle through the liver until a bile duct is located, then opacifying the biliary system with iodinated contrast.

Structural Abnormalities

Multiple congenital anomalies and variants of the gallbladder and biliary tree are possible. With a few exceptions, these anomalies usually are asymptomatic and are incidental findings at a later stage in the patient's life.

Gallbladder developmental anomalies encompass a spectrum ranging from agenesis to hypoplasia. **Gallbladder agenesis** is associated with other anomalies, including rectovaginal fistula, congenital heart disease, imperforate anus, polysplenia, and absence of one or more bones. Agenesis of the gallbladder is an infrequent cause of nonvisualization of the gallbladder on oral cholecystogram, hepatobiliary scan, or ultrasound. **Gallbladder hypoplasia** is associated with cystic fibrosis. The patient may have biliary

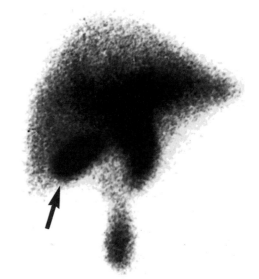

Figure 9–5. Normal hepatobiliary scan. A nuclear medicine hepatobiliary scan performed with ^{99m}Tc-IDA allows prompt visualization of the gallbladder *(arrow)* as well as biliary ductal and small bowel activity.

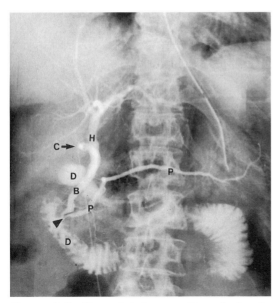

Figure 9–6. Normal intraoperative cholangiogram. Normal biliary and pancreatic ductal anatomy is delineated by injection of contrast through the cystic duct remnant during an intraoperative cholangiogram: common hepatic duct (H), cystic duct remnant (C), common bile duct (B), major papilla *(arrowhead)*, main pancreatic duct (P), and duodenum (D). (From Mettler FA: Essentials of Radiology. Philadephia, WB Saunders, 1995, p 200.)

colic or extrahepatic biliary calculi or may be asymptomatic.

Gallbladder duplication is a rare anomaly resulting from a persistent longitudinal septum. Two separate lumens with two cystic ducts define duplication, whereas two lumens with a shared cystic duct define a **bifid gallbladder.**

Abnormal locations of the gallbladder occur with situs inversus or as an isolated finding. The gallbladder may be left-sided or midline, intrahepatic, suprahepatic, in the falciform ligament, in the anterior abdominal wall, in the transverse mesocolon, or posterior near the spine. A **floating gallbladder** occurs when the gallbladder mesentery is long. The gallbladder then moves with changes in patient position and may herniate through the foramen of Winslow into the lesser sac. Ultrasound and CT are nonspecific, identifying a cystic structure in the lesser sac.

Gallbladder torsion presents similar to acute cholecystitis and occurs when the gallbladder mesentery is long or when there are no mesenteric attachments to stabilize the gallbladder. Large stones in the gallbladder fundus may predispose the gallbladder to torsion by lengthening the mesentery. On ultrasound and CT, a thickened, distended gallbladder may be identified, but the finding is nonspecific. Gangrene may develop with prolonged torsion.

Biliary tract anomalies are found in 2.4% of autopsies and 5% to 13% of intraoperative cholangiograms. The most common anomaly is an aberrant intrahepatic duct that drains a portion of the liver into the common hepatic duct, common bile duct, right hepatic duct, cystic duct, or gallbladder itself. This anomalous duct may be injured during cholecystectomy if it is not identified properly.

Choledochal cysts are congenital dilations of the extrahepatic bile ducts. This is the most common congenital bile duct anomaly and often is associated with other gallbladder anomalies, biliary stenosis or atresia, and congenital hepatic fibrosis. Clinical presentation usually occurs before 10 years of age but can present in adulthood as well. Presenting symptoms include obstructive jaundice in the neonate and right upper quadrant pain with intermittent jaundice and fever in older children and adults. Complications are numerous and include rupture with secondary bile peritonitis, cholangitis, calculus formation, portal vein thrombosis, malignant transformation to cholangiocarcinoma, recurrent pancreatitis, and biliary cirrhosis with portal hypertension. Treatment involves surgical resection.

The choledochal cyst is diagnosed with cholangiography as a cystic collection of contrast material in communication with the bile duct. There may be fusiform dilation of the common bile duct (type I) (Fig. 9–7A) or a saccular outpouching from the duct (type II) (Fig. 9–7B). These cysts also may be visualized with ultrasound and CT. On ultrasound and CT, a cystic fluid-filled structure that communicates with the biliary system is visualized inferior to the porta hepatis. This is a nonspecific appearance that could represent a hepatic cyst, pancreatic pseudocyst, or enteric duplication cyst. To differentiate these entities, a hepatobiliary scan may be performed. Findings include an area of decreased activity within the liver that later fills and has prolonged activity as a result of stasis. Radiographs may show a right upper quadrant mass displacing the right kidney. An upper gastrointestinal exam-

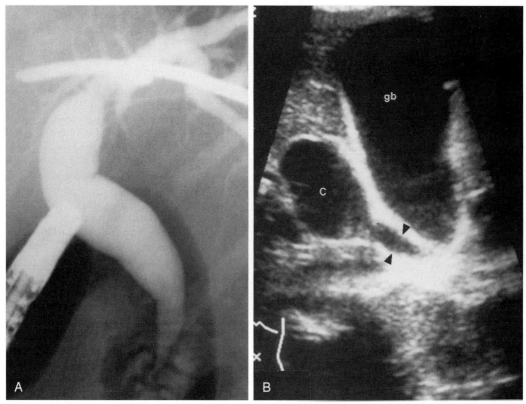

Figure 9–7. Choledochal cysts. A, ERCP demonstrates fusiform dilation of the common bile duct from a type I choledochal cyst. **B,** Sonogram reveals a saccular outpouching of the common bile duct from a type II choledochal cyst (c), with a normal-caliber distal duct *(arrowheads)*. The gallbladder (gb) is visualized to the left of the choledochal cyst.

ination may show widening of the duodenal sweep.

A **choledochocele** (a form of choledochal cyst) is a rare anomaly involving a dilated portion of the distal common bile duct that protrudes into the duodenum. This anomaly may be congenital or may be acquired after passage of gallstones with resultant inflammation. Most commonly, the common bile duct drains into the cyst, which then drains into the duodenum. Alternatively the cyst may drain into the adjacent intramural common bile duct.

Presenting symptoms are similar to those of the choledochal cyst and include biliary colic and episodic jaundice. Gallstones and sludge often are present. On barium studies, there is a well-defined duodenal filling defect in the region of the papilla that changes with compression and peristalsis. The choledochocele does not fill with barium, in contrast to intraluminal diverticula. Cholangiography reveals smooth clublike dilation of the intramural common bile duct segment.

Caroli disease, also known as *communicating cavernous ectasia of biliary ducts,* is a rare disorder characterized by segmental saccular dilation of intrahepatic bile ducts. Caroli disease most commonly presents in adulthood with right upper quadrant pain, intermittent fever, and jaundice. This disease is associated with medullary sponge kidney and infantile polycystic kidney disease.

Cholangiography shows saccular dilations with stones, strictures, and communicating hepatic abscesses (Fig. 9–8). On CT, the "central dot" sign is caused by visualization of a bright contrast-enhancing dot surrounded by a fluid density. This dot represents the intraluminal portal vein within a dilated duct. CT and ultrasound show multiple cystic areas within the liver. Hepatobiliary scans show areas of decreased activity that fill in on later images. Patients with Caroli disease may develop bile stasis with recurrent cholangitis, liver abscesses, or septicemia. There is an increased risk for

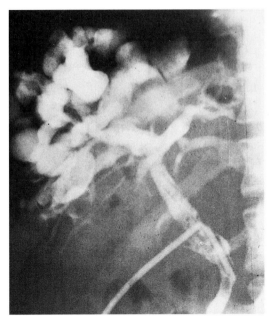

Figure 9–8. Caroli disease. T-tube cholangiogram reveals marked saccular dilation of the intrahepatic bile ducts.

cholangiocarcinoma. Palliative treatment involves antibiotics, biliary drainage, and stone removal, but overall prognosis is poor.

Diseases of the Gallbladder and Bile Ducts

Cholelithiasis is a common disorder affecting many adults in the United States, women much more commonly than men. Other predisposing factors include obesity, increasing age, elevated triglycerides, hyperalimentation, ileal intestinal disease, diabetes mellitus, pregnancy, and Native American heritage. Most patients with gallstones are asymptomatic, but those who have symptoms may experience nausea, right upper quadrant pain, and postprandial colic. These patients have a 1% to 2% per year risk of progression to acute cholecystitis.

In the United States, most **gallstones** are composed of cholesterol and lesser amounts of lecithin and bile salts such as calcium carbonate. These stones are radiolucent on conventional radiographs 85% of the time. Pigmented stones contain calcium bilirubinate and are more likely to be seen on radiographs (Fig. 9–9A). Filling defects are seen with oral cholecystography (Fig. 9–9B). On ultrasound, a stone appears as an echo-

genic focus with posterior acoustical shadowing (Fig. 9–9C). The gallstones must be mobile and layer dependently in more than one position. Decubitus and upright views are useful in this respect. Small stones in the range of several millimeters may not shadow. If the gallbladder is fibrotic and contracted and contains multiple stones, a *double arc shadow* may be seen. This shadow consists of two parallel echogenic lines representing the gallbladder wall and the stone with a lucent rim interposed representing the narrowed lumen.

Biliary sludge is associated with bile stasis and can be seen in the gallbladder on ultrasound. Sludge is echogenic but does not shadow unless it also contains stones. Sludge may form clumps that move slowly with changes in position. This is known as **tumefactive sludge.** Mobility must be shown to exclude a mass lesion within the gallbladder.

Mirizzi syndrome is caused by gallstone impaction in the gallbladder infundibulum or cystic duct. This impaction leads to inflammation and possible erosion of the stone into the common hepatic duct. Inflammation produces mechanical obstruction of the adjacent common hepatic duct and dilation of the biliary system proximally. The dilated ducts may be visualized with ultrasonography or CT.

Another possible complication is **gallstone ileus** (a misnomer). This complication occurs in the setting of chronic cholecystitis when a large gallstone, usually greater than 2 cm in diameter, erodes into the duodenum and causes a mechanical small bowel obstruction, usually in the terminal ileum. On conventional radiographs, biliary air, small bowel obstruction, or an ectopic calcified gallstone may be visualized. A barium gastrointestinal study may identify the biliary-enteric fistula. Gallstones may erode into the stomach, colon, or peritoneal cavity.

Acute cholecystitis occurs when the cystic duct becomes obstructed by an impacted stone. This condition usually is seen in patients with chronic biliary symptoms. Stone impaction leads to local inflammation, gallbladder distention, gallbladder wall edema, and eventual necrosis. Most of these attacks remit with spontaneous passage of the obstructing stone.

Findings consistent with acute cholecystitis on ultrasound include cholelithiasis with associated gallbladder wall thickening, gall-

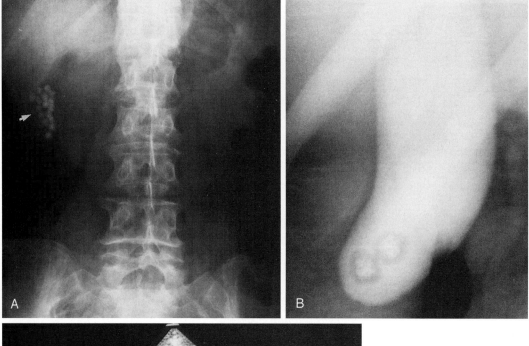

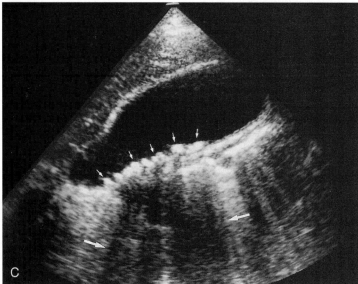

Figure 9–9. Cholelithiasis. Gallstones can be visualized on various imaging modalities: **A,** A conventional radiograph of the abdomen demonstrates calcified gallstones in the right upper quadrant *(arrow).* **B,** Oral cholecystogram illustrates two gallstones with central calcifications layering dependently in the opacified gallbladder. **C,** Longitudinal sonogram of the gallbladder reveals multiple gallstones as echogenic foci *(small arrows)* with posterior acoustical shadowing (outlined by *large arrows*).

bladder distention, and the sonographic Murphy sign. A **sonographic Murphy sign** is present when there is maximal pain over the gallbladder when this region is compressed by the ultrasound transducer. The gallbladder wall should not measure greater than 3 mm in thickness. Edema within the wall may be seen as a sonolucent middle layer (Fig. 9–10). Gallbladder wall thickening is not specific to acute cholecystitis because this thickening also occurs with hypoalbuminemia, hepatitis, and sepsis.

Hepatobiliary scanning is more sensitive than sonography in detecting acute cholecystitis. The radionuclide usually accumulates in the gallbladder 30 minutes after intravenous injection. If the cystic duct is obstructed, the gallbladder is not visualized (Fig. 9–11). If the gallbladder is visualized on delayed films at 4 hours, the diagnosis of **chronic cholecystitis** can be made.

Emphysematous cholecystitis is a severe condition most commonly seen in diabetics and other debilitated patients. More common in men, emphysematous cholecystitis is thought to be the sequela of gallbladder

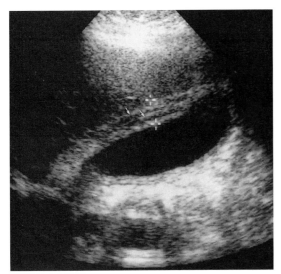

Figure 9–10. Gallbladder wall edema. Longitudinal sonogram demonstrates a thickened gallbladder wall (between calipers) with hypoechoic striations *(arrows)* from mural edema.

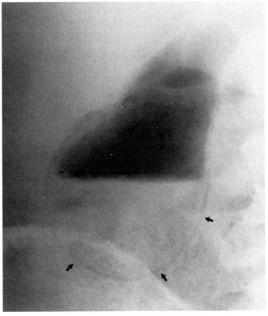

Figure 9–12. Emphysematous cholecystitis. Conventional radiograph demonstrates a gas-bile level in the gallbladder lumen as well as gas in the gallbladder wall *(arrows).*

ischemia with secondary infection by *Clostridia, Escherichia coli, Staphylococcus,* or *Streptococcus.* Gas in the gallbladder lumen may be seen on conventional radiographs (Fig. 9–12). On ultrasound, bright echoes are visualized with "dirty" or poorly defined posterior shadows in the wall or lumen (calcification produces "clean" posterior shad-ows). The risk of perforation is increased in these patients and usually warrants emergent cholecystectomy.

Complications of acute cholecystitis include gangrenous cholecystitis and perfora-

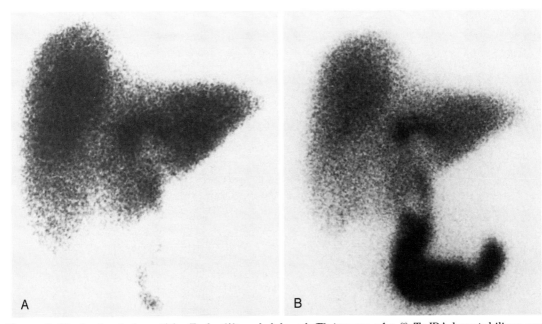

Figure 9–11. Acute cholecystitis. Early **(A)** and delayed **(B)** images of a ^{99m}Tc-IDA hepatobiliary scan display persistent failure of visualization of the gallbladder.

tion. **Gangrenous cholecystitis,** representing mural necrosis, can be diagnosed with ultrasound or hepatobiliary scanning. On ultrasonography, shaggy asymmetry in the wall and coarse intraluminal echoes representing intraluminal hemorrhage and membranes may be identified. These intraluminal echoes are nondependent and correspond to fibrinous exudate and sloughed mucosa. On hepatobiliary scan, a faint rim of increased pericholecystic activity secondary to hyperemia may be present.

Perforation occurs in less than 20% of acute cholecystitis cases. Most are subacute and encapsulate, forming **pericholecystic abscesses;** this may be seen on ultrasound or CT as a pericholecystic fluid collection (Fig. 9–13). Hepatobiliary imaging may reveal extravasated radionuclide, unless the cystic duct is obstructed. If the duct is obstructed, the radionuclide cannot enter the gallbladder.

Acalculous cholecystitis is seen in approximately 5% to 10% of acute cholecystitis cases. Altered gallbladder function with decreased motility is most likely responsible. This altered function can be seen in patients with starvation, burns, hyperalimentation, or shock. Inflammation, infection with *Salmonella* (salmonellosis) or *Vibrio cholerae* (cholera), and extrinsic compression of the cystic duct by neoplasm or lymphadenopathy are other possible causes. In patients with acquired immunodeficiency syndrome (AIDS), acalculous cholecystitis is associated with infection by many organisms, including cytomegalovirus, *Cryptosporidium, Microsporidium,* and *Mycobacterium avium-intracellulare.* Signs and symptoms are identical to acute cholecystitis caused by gallstones. With ultrasonography, it is important to search for gallbladder wall thickening and gallbladder distention in the absence of calculi. Pericholecystic fluid may be seen. Nonvisualization of the gallbladder secondary to cystic duct edema may be identified on hepatobiliary scan.

Chronic cholecystitis, whether stone-related or acalculous, is more common than the acute form. Gallstones and a thickened gallbladder wall are identified on ultrasound. With hepatobiliary scanning, the gallbladder may be visualized on delayed images (1 to 4 hours), with visualization of the bowel occurring before gallbladder visualization. The patient is asymptomatic until the cystic duct becomes obstructed and acute inflammation is superimposed.

Porcelain gallbladder is a gross pathologic descriptive term that refers to blue discoloration and fragile consistency of a gallbladder wall that has become calcified from chronic inflammation. Gallstones are present in most cases. The calcified wall is seen readily on radiographs and CT with the periphery more densely calcified (Fig. 9–14). The gallbladder is nonfunctioning and nonvisualized with cholecystography. With ultrasound, there may be multiple clumps of echoes with posterior shadowing or an echogenic shadowing curvilinear structure. Alternatively the wall may be echogenic with

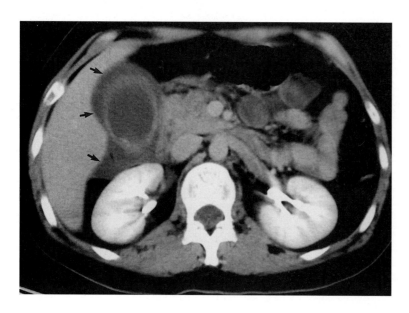

Figure 9–13. Pericholecystic fluid. Contrasted CT scan reveals low-attenuation fluid *(arrows)* surrounding the gallbladder. The gallbladder wall is thickened.

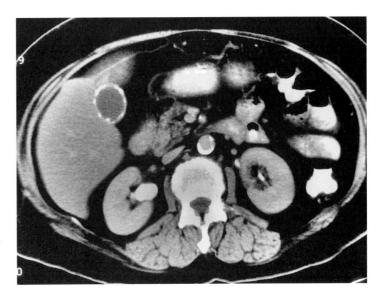

Figure 9–14. Calcified gallbladder. Contrasted CT indicates concentric calcification of gallbladder wall in a patient diagnosed with porcelain gallbladder.

little posterior shadowing, which may simulate emphysematous cholecystitis. The disease usually is asymptomatic and is five times more common in women than in men. The risk of gallbladder carcinoma is increased to approximately 25% so that cholecystectomy usually is performed prophylactically.

Milk of calcium bile is bile containing precipitated calcium salts that occurs in the setting of chronic cholecystitis. On conventional radiographs, the gallbladder appears diffusely opaque. The gallbladder is nonfunctional on oral cholecystography. The bile is echogenic and appears similar to sludge with multiple echogenic gallstones on ultrasound. There usually is a fluid-fluid level, with bile layering on top of the milk of calcium bile.

Choledocholithiasis in the United States is most commonly the result of gallstones passed from the gallbladder. This is the most common cause of bile duct obstruction and may cause recurrent jaundice and biliary colic. Chills and fever may be present if cholangitis develops. Alternatively, patients may remain asymptomatic and pass stones less than 6 mm in diameter spontaneously. Of cholecystectomy patients, 12% to 15% have common bile duct stones. Common duct stone prevalence increases with age.

Primary duct stones form within the ducts, usually owing to bacterial deconjugation of bilirubin. This deconjugation may be enhanced by biliary stasis, bacterial infection with gram-negative enteric organisms, or parasitic infection with *Clonorchis* and *As-*

caris. Parasitic infection is an uncommon cause in the United States.

Similar to gallstones, common bile duct stones may be seen as filling defects with ERCP and intraoperative and postoperative cholangiography. Filling defects that may mimic stones include injected air bubbles, blood clots, debris, and mucus (Fig. 9–15*A*). Air bubbles tend to rise, whereas stones settle dependently. ERCP is advantageous because stones may be extracted with or without sphincterotomy, and biliary stents may be placed.

Ultrasonography is less specific, but common duct stones can be visualized in 55% to 75% of patients. Distal common bile duct stones may be missed, however. The appearance of small shadowing echogenic foci is typical (Fig. 9–15*B*), but posterior acoustic shadows may not be seen in approximately 10% of stones because of their small size. Other lesions may have this appearance, including blood clots, sludge, and infection. The patient may be scanned before and after ingesting a fatty meal. The dietary fats cause the release of cholecystokinin, which increases bile flow and relaxes the sphincter of Oddi. If the common bile duct is obstructed, an increase in diameter of greater than 2 mm occurs. Additional scanning following a fatty meal is especially helpful in patients who are postcholecystectomy, with an enlarged duct at baseline.

On CT, stones may contain enough calcium to be visualized as high-attenuation foci with or without common bile duct dilation. The "target" sign shows a rounded den-

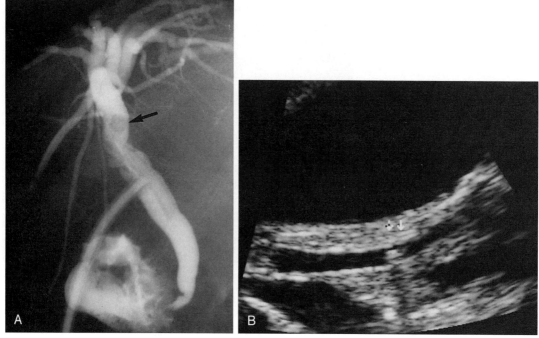

Figure 9–15. Choledocholithiasis. A, T-tube cholangiogram after cholecystectomy reveals a faceted radiolucent filling defect *(arrow)* in the common hepatic duct, representing a retained stone. Note the dilation of the intrahepatic biliary tree. **B,** Longitudinal sonogram of the common bile duct allows visualization of an echogenic stone *(arrows),* with posterior acoustical shadowing.

sity (the stone) surrounded by a ring of water-density bile. Hepatobiliary scanning is less helpful and may show only prominent ducts with delayed activity in the duodenum. Magnetic resonance cholangiography has increasing utility in the detection of common bile duct stones with similar sensitivity to ERCP and without the risk of contrast administration or radiation.

Biliary Inflammation and Infection

Acute cholangitis is characterized by right upper quadrant pain, fever, chills, and jaundice, which usually is caused by bacterial infection, typically by *E. coli.* Biliary stasis secondary to choledocholithiasis, post-surgical stricture, and papillary stenosis predisposes to infection. Other less common causes include cholangiocarcinoma, pancreatic carcinoma, and malignant periportal lymphadenopathy. In patients with AIDS, cholangitis often is related to infection with cytomegalovirus, *M. avium-intracellulare, Cryptosporidium,* and *Microsporidium.* Acute cholangitis may subside owing to spontane-

ous relief of the obstruction, but it may progress to **suppurative cholangitis,** with accumulation of purulent material in the biliary ducts. Complications of suppurative cholangitis include septicemia, shock, and miliary hepatic abscess formation. Suppurative cholangitis carries a high mortality rate and requires prompt decompression.

Ultrasound may show dilated ducts containing echogenic material, and CT shows high-attenuation material within dilated ducts. ERCP and PTC can show filling defects within the biliary tree.

Abscesses can be identified as contrast collections that fill from dilated bile ducts on cholangiography. AIDS-related cholangitis frequently shows distal common bile duct stricture with a dilated extrahepatic ductal system as well as multiple stricures, diverticula, and pruning of the intrahepatic bile ducts similar to that seen in sclerosing cholangitis.

Recurrent pyogenic cholangitis, also known as **Oriental cholangiohepatitis,** is endemic in certain Asian populations. Recurrent pyogenic cholangitis is thought to be caused by parasitic infestation with the liver flukes *Clonorchis sinensis* and *Opisthorchis*

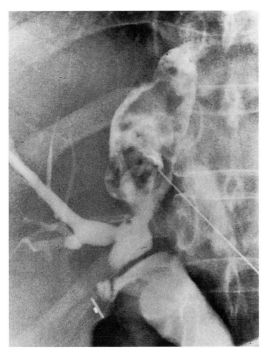

Figure 9–16. Recurrent pyogenic cholangitis. ERCP demonstrates dilated intrahepatic ducts with irregular filling defects affecting the left-sided system as well as the common bile duct.

viverrini and the roundworm *Ascaris lumbricoides.* Infestation leads to biliary stasis and secondary infection by enteric organisms. The gram-negative bacteria then deconjugate the bilirubin and cause pigment stone formation. Recurrent pyogenic cholangitis presents in a similar fashion to acute cholangitis with right upper quadrant pain, jaundice, fever, and chills. Multiple exacerbations and remissions occur with eventual duct injury and biliary cirrhosis. Sonography and CT identify dilated intrahepatic and extrahepatic ducts containing stones and sludge (Fig. 9–16). The lateral segment of the left lobe is involved most commonly.

Pneumobilia may occur secondary to gas-forming organisms or a patulous sphincter of Oddi. On ultrasonography, echoes with shadowing may represent air or stones within the bile ducts, and CT differentiates these findings. Segmental hepatic atrophy may be seen on CT as well. ERCP and PTC show decreased branching of the intrahepatic biliary tree, dilated ducts, smooth strictures, and filling defects compatible with stones. Ascariasis and other parasitic infestations may cause biliary obstruction and an inflammatory response. These

worms may be seen as tubular filling defects on ERCP or PTC.

Primary sclerosing cholangitis is a disease primarily affecting young men. Although associated with ulcerative colitis, the underlying cause is unknown. **Secondary sclerosing cholangitis** may be associated with pancreatitis, mediastinal or retroperitoneal fibrosis, thyroiditis, and Peyronie disease. These patients present with jaundice, fatigue, pruritus, and right upper quadrant pain. Prognosis is poor and correlates with the degree of stricturing.

Cholangiography identifies multifocal strictures, especially involving bifurcations. Normal segments of bile duct are interposed between strictured segments, giving the ducts a beaded appearance. With progression of the disease, longer strictures and pruning of the peripheral ducts may occur (Fig. 9–17). In the extrahepatic ducts, small diverticular outpouchings rarely are seen. These diverticula are nonspecific, however, and may be seen with other biliary abnormalities. On ultrasound, the ducts appear brightly echogenic owing to the wall thick-

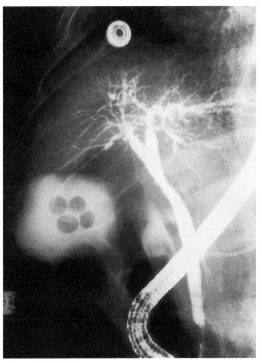

Figure 9–17. Sclerosing cholangitis. ERCP reveals an irregular, beaded appearance of the intrahepatic bile ducts. Four radiolucent gallstones appear as filling defects in the opacified gallbladder.

ening, and common bile duct wall thickening may be seen. With sonography and CT, irregular intrahepatic biliary dilation is seen; however, failure to visualize the ducts because of sclerosis is more common. Hepatobiliary scans show patchy hepatic activity with persistent areas of activity in intrahepatic biliary tree locations. These findings are not specific, and cholangiocarcinoma must be included in the differential diagnosis.

Papillary stenosis (biliary dyskinesia) may be primary or secondary. Primary stenosis occurs in only 10% of cases and is caused by congenital malformation of the papilla, postinflammatory changes, or adenomyomatosis. Secondary stenosis may be the result of prior stone passage, functional stenosis from pancreatic disorders including pancreas divisum or pancreatitis, reflex spasm, previous surgery, or periampullary neoplasm. Ampullary stenosis also may be seen with AIDS-related cholangitis.

Symptoms of papillary stenosis are similar to those of choledocholithiasis, with right upper quadrant pain and laboratory evidence of cholestasis. On ultrasound, there may be dilation of the common bile duct and sometimes the pancreatic duct (Fig. 9–18). With hepatobiliary scanning, there is delayed radionuclide transport from the bile ducts into the small bowel of greater than 45 minutes. ERCP is useful for direct visualization of the papilla with concurrent biopsy. Manometry can be performed with the endoscope to evaluate for functional stenosis.

Treatment involves endoscopic sphincterotomy.

The term ***hyperplastic cholecystoses*** has been used to describe benign noninflammatory gallbladder anomalies that involve hyperplasia of components of the gallbladder wall. The two best described are adenomyomatosis and cholesterolosis. Both conditions are more common in women and are seen in 5% to 25% of surgically removed gallbladders. Patients may be asymptomatic or may present with biliary colic.

In **adenomyomatosis,** there is marked thickening of the gallbladder wall with **Rokitansky-Aschoff** sinuses, which are pronounced infoldings of the epithelial lining. These sinuses become surrounded by the thickened muscle and may fill on oral cholecystography, appearing as multiple tiny extraluminal collections of contrast. Adenomyomatosis may involve the entire gallbladder wall or may be more focal. Alternatively the process may be limited to the gallbladder fundus, giving a sessile mass known as an **adenomyoma.** Ultrasound may show a thickened wall with small anechoic spaces representing the sinuses. If the sinuses are filled with debris, they appear echogenic and have V-shaped ring-down artifacts (Fig. 9–19).

CT shows wall thickening, but this is nonspecific. Included in the differential diagnosis are gallbladder carcinoma and acute or chronic cholecystitis. Gallstones are associated with carcinoma and cholecystitis so that the absence of stones may suggest adenomyomatosis. Also, gallbladder carci-

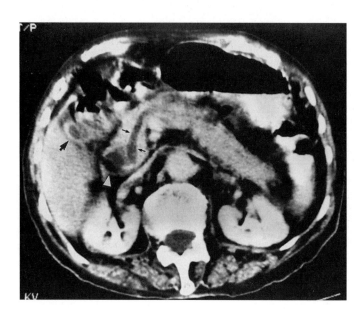

Figure 9–18. Papillary stenosis. Contrasted CT indicates a dilated pancreatic duct *(small black arrows)* and dilated common bile duct *(white arrowhead).* Also note the small contracted gallbladder *(large black arrow).*

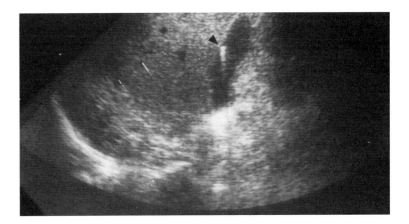

Figure 9–19. Adenomyomatosis. Longitudinal sonogram of the gallbladder demonstrates a V-shaped echogenic ring-down artifact from a debris-filled Rokitansky-Aschoff sinus *(arrowhead).*

noma–associated wall thickening is usually more irregular, and invasion of adjacent structures excludes adenomyomatosis.

Cholesterolosis is a condition consisting of abnormal deposition of cholesterol esters in the subepithelial tissue of the gallbladder wall. There is no demonstrable relationship to serum or bile cholesterol levels or to cholesterol gallstones. Two forms of cholesterolosis exist: the planar form and the cholesterol polyp. In the planar form, the gallbladder wall is involved diffusely. On gross inspection, the tiny yellow cholesterol-containing nodules, when seen on an inflamed background, resemble a strawberry, giving the name "strawberry" gallbladder. This planar form is not detectable radiographically. A more focal form, the **cholesterol polyp,** is more common. The cholesterol polyps are approximately 1 cm in diameter and may be single or multiple. On oral cholecystogram, these polyps appear as fixed filling defects. By ultrasonography, these are small fixed echogenic foci that do not cause posterior shadowing (Fig. 9–20). Conditions to include in the differential diagnosis of multiple masses include adenoma, papilloma, carcinoids, or metastases.

Benign and Malignant Neoplasms

Benign gallbladder tumors are rare and are found incidentally at cholecystectomy. Gallbladder **polyps** may be seen as fixed, nondependent, filling defects on oral cholecystogram. On ultrasound, they are nonmobile, echogenic masses adherent to the gallbladder wall. These polyps usually do not shadow, which helps differentiate them from

gallstones. Most of these are cholesterol polyps or adenomas.

Adenomas usually are solitary lesions that may be sessile or pedunculated. These lesions have the same appearance as the cholesterol polyps on oral cholecystogram and ultrasound. Most believe that the gallbladder adenoma has a low risk of malignant transformation.

Other rare benign tumors include leiomyoma, fibroma, lipoma, and hemangioma. Heterotopic gastric and pancreatic tissue also can occur in the gallbladder.

Benign tumors of the extrahepatic biliary tree are uncommon. **Biliary cystadenoma** is similar to ovarian and pancreatic cystadeno-

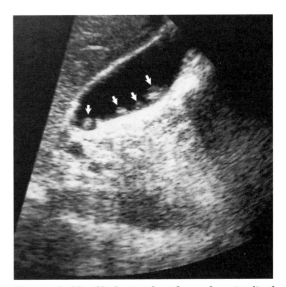

Figure 9–20. Cholesterol polyps. Longitudinal sonogram of the gallbladder shows echogenic foci *(arrows)* that do not have posterior acoustic shadows and remain fixed to the wall during the examination.

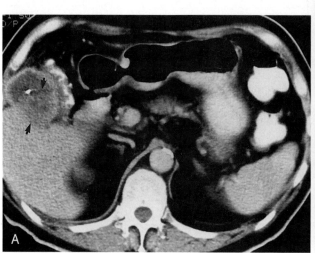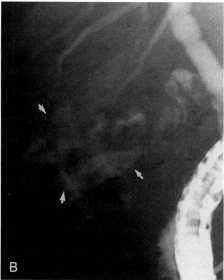

Figure 9–21. Gallbladder carcinoma. A, Contrasted CT through the gallbladder shows a soft tissue mass replacing the gallbladder lumen *(arrows)*. The small high attenuation focus within the gallbladder represents a gallstone. **B,** ERCP illustrates irregular filling defects in the gallbladder *(arrows)*, from a mass occupying the lumen.

mas. These tumors are more common in middle-aged women. The appearance is that of a complex cystic mass with septa that may calcify. The mass is water density on CT and hypoechoic on ultrasound. These lesions are more common in an intrahepatic location. If they do occur in an extrahepatic location, biliary dilation may be identified. **Biliary cystadenocarcinoma** is the malignant form of this lesion and appears similar to the benign form on imaging.

Adenomas, hamartomas, fibromas, lipomas, and heterotopic gastric and pancreatic tissue can be found in the biliary tree as well. If these masses become large enough, biliary obstruction and dilation occur.

Gallbladder carcinoma is the fifth most common gastrointestinal malignancy after colorectal, pancreatic, gastric, and esophageal carcinomas. Gallbladder carcinoma is three to four times more common in women and usually affects patients aged 60 to 70. Of gallbladder carcinoma patients, 75% have cholelithiasis, suggesting chronic irritation as a contributory factor. Having a calcified gallbladder dramatically increases the risk of malignancy. Most patients have cholecystitis symptoms, including right upper quadrant pain, nausea, jaundice, or weight loss.

Most malignancies of the gallbladder are primary **adenocarcinoma. Squamous cell carcinoma** and **anaplastic carcinoma** are less common. A scirrhous type of adenocarcinoma infiltrates the wall and eventually fills the lumen. Metastasis by extension along the biliary tree as well as by lymphatic spread is common at the time of diagnosis, making prognosis poor despite surgical excision.

On sonography and CT, there are several presentations of gallbladder carcinoma (Fig. 9–21). There may be an inhomogeneous hypoechoic or low-density mass that obscures the gallbladder margins and replaces the lumen. The mass usually enhances on a contrasted CT scan. Invasion into the liver is suggestive of carcinoma. This appearance may be confused, however, with cholecystitis complicated by pericholecystic abscess. Another pattern seen on ultrasound is focal or diffuse wall thickening. As opposed to cholecystitis-associated wall thickening, carcinoma usually causes asymmetric and irregular thickening. Other clues to making a diagnosis of carcinoma include finding an associated mass, lymphadenopathy, and hepatic invasion. The third and least common radiographic presentation is that of a fixed polypoid mass projecting into the gallbladder lumen that does not produce acoustic shadows. **Metastases** to the gallbladder most commonly originate from melanoma and may mimic primary gallbladder carcinoma.

Cholangiocarcinoma is the main malignancy of the biliary ducts but is an uncommon lesion. This neoplasm is an adenocarcinoma arising from bile duct epithelium and may occur in intrahepatic or extrahepatic biliary ducts. When the mass occurs at the bifurcation of the common hepatic duct, the eponym *Klatskin tumor* is given to this lesion. Men are affected more commonly than women, usually between the ages of 60 and 70. Predisposing factors include sclerosing cholangitis, ulcerative colitis, choledochal cyst, and *Clonorchis* infection. Signs and symptoms include weight loss, jaundice, pruritus, and anorexia. Patients rarely present with symptoms of cholangitis.

Klatskin tumor is the most common extrahepatic cholangiocarcinoma. Biliary dilation proximal to the stricturing lesion may be seen on ultrasound, CT, or cholangiography (Fig. 9–22). On ultrasound and CT, it may be difficult to show a mass or wall thickening; however, an abrupt transition between normal and narrowed biliary duct is suggestive of tumor. A tapered narrowing is more characteristic of a benign stricture. CT is more sensitive for showing a mass lesion that may be high or low attenuation and may enhance with contrast administration, especially on delayed images. Similar to gallbladder carcinoma, additional findings that suggest malignancy include hepatic invasion and regional lymphadenopathy. CT scan shows hepatic lobar atrophy with dilation of the biliary tree supplying that segment. Distal common bile duct cholangiocarcinomas usually are smaller tumors that may appear as a stricture or polypoid mass. Treatment involves surgical resection, stenting, and liver transplantation.

Periampullary carcinomas arise at the ampulla of Vater and originate from bile duct, pancreas, or duodenum. Biliary dilation is seen proximal to these polypoid lesions. **Biliary cystadenocarcinoma** appears similar to the benign cystadenoma and was mentioned briefly earlier. Other rare neoplasms include lymphoma, leiomyosarcoma, carcinoid, and metastases from lung, breast, other gastrointestinal malignancies, and malignant melanoma.

Miscellaneous Conditions

Surgical or endoscopic manipulation of the biliary tract is common and may lead to various complications. A **bile leak** may be the result of iatrogenic bile duct injury, improperly placed T-tubes, or blockage of the distal common bile duct by retained stones or blood clot. This leak may cause bile peritonitis, which carries a high mortality rate. On CT, there is ascites with diffuse inflammatory changes. The presence, but not the actual size, of a bile leak is diagnosed easily with a hepatobiliary scan showing activity in an aberrant location (Fig. 9–23A). Cholangiography also shows the leak. A **biloma** is a focal collection that develops. Ultrasound shows a hypoechoic cystic structure in a subhepatic location. CT shows a low-attenuation cystic lesion (Fig. 9–23B). Hematoma

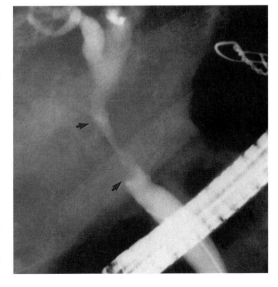

Figure 9–22. Cholangiocarcinoma. ERCP demonstrates an irregular stricture (between *arrows*) at the bifurcation of the common hepatic duct from a Klatskin tumor.

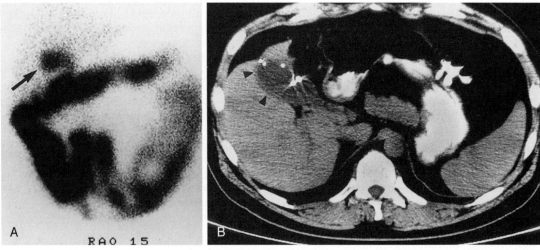

Figure 9–23. Biloma. A, Hepatobiliary scan reveals a focal collection of activity *(arrow)* in the expected location of the gallbladder, consistent with a postoperative biloma. **B,** Noncontrasted CT in the same patient shows a right upper quadrant fluid collection *(arrowheads),* also representing the biloma. High-attenuation foci represent surgical clips.

and abscess are other complications after surgery or trauma that can be identified on ultrasound and CT.

Postoperative ductal stricture can occur if the bile duct walls are damaged leading to fibrosis and scarring. These strictures are identified with cholangiography and usually can be stented with good result. Biliary-enteric and biliary-venous fistulas are other iatrogenic complications that can be diagnosed with cholangiography. Barium studies show filling of the biliary tree at the site of the biliary-enteric fistula.

Retained calculi are seen in 2% to 5% of patients after cholecystectomy. Sphincterotomy and endoscopic stone extraction are successful in treating this complication.

Although the biliary system is affected rarely, blunt abdominal **trauma** may result in gallbladder perforation, contusion, or avulsion with resultant necrosis. **Acute hemorrhagic cholecystitis** may develop when intraluminal clots block the cystic duct. Penetrating trauma, similar to iatrogenic injury, may result in bile duct transection with biloma formation.

Suggested Readings

Berk RB, Ferrucci JT Jr, Leopold GR: Radiology of the Gallbladder and Bile Ducts: Diagnosis and Intervention. Philadelphia, WB Saunders, 1983.

Friedman AC, Dachman AH: Radiology of the Liver, Biliary Tract, and Pancreas, 2nd ed. St. Louis, Mosby-Year Book, 1994.

Gore RM, Levine MS, Laufer I: Textbook of Gastrointestinal Radiology, 2nd ed. Philadelphia, WB Saunders, 2000.

TEN

Pancreas

JEFFREY D. HOUSTON, M.D., AND MICHAEL DAVIS, M.D.

Normal Anatomy

The pancreas is located in the anterior pararenal space of the retroperitoneum and has a complex anatomic relationship with the adjacent abdominal viscera. It is bounded anteriorly by the lesser peritoneal sac, posteriorly by the great vessels and splenic vein, and laterally by the duodenal C-loop and spleen. The organ spans 12 to 15 cm transversely and is divided into the uncinate process, head, neck, body, and tail (Fig. 10–1). Normal anteroposterior measurement of the head is 3 cm, with the body and tail tapering toward the splenic hilum, measuring 2.5 cm and 2 cm. The uncinate process is positioned between the inferior vena cava and the superior mesenteric vein, just before the superior mesenteric vein unites with the splenic vein to form the portal vein. The superior mesenteric vein anatomically separates the pancreatic head and body, and the left lateral border of the lumbar spine demarcates the body and tail.

Main and accessory pancreatic ducts provide exocrine drainage for the gland (Fig. 10–2). The **main pancreatic duct** (of Wirsung) normally courses from the pancreatic tail, through the body, and into the head, where it unites with the common bile duct to form the **ampulla of Vater.** The ampulla is surrounded by the musculature of the **sphincter of Oddi,** which promotes drainage into the second portion of the duodenum at the **major papilla.** The **accessory pancreatic duct** (of Santorini) communicates with the main pancreatic duct in the head and drains through the **minor papilla,** located slightly

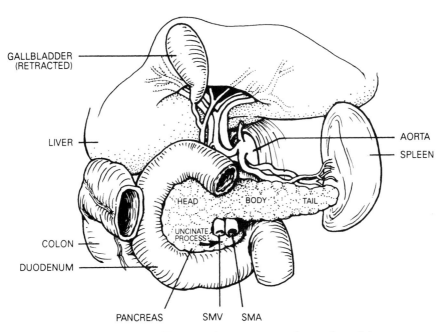

Figure 10–1. Anatomy of the pancreas. The complex anatomic relationship of the pancreas to adjacent structures: superior mesenteric vein (SMV), superior mesenteric artery (SMA).

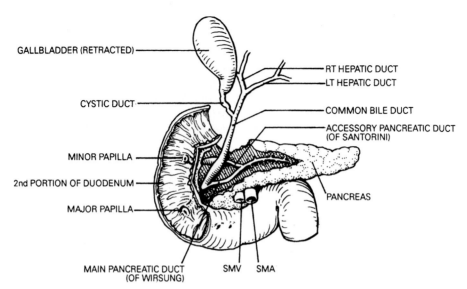

GALLBLADDER (RETRACTED)

RT HEPATIC DUCT
LT HEPATIC DUCT

CYSTIC DUCT

COMMON BILE DUCT

ACCESSORY PANCREATIC DUCT
(OF SANTORINI)

MINOR PAPILLA

2nd PORTION OF DUODENUM

PANCREAS

MAJOR PAPILLA

MAIN PANCREATIC DUCT   SMV   SMA
(OF WIRSUNG)

Figure 10–2. Pancreatic ductal anatomy. The normal pancreatic ductal anatomy and its relationship to the duodenum: superior mesenteric vein (SMV), superior mesenteric artery (SMA).

cephalad and anteromedial to the major papilla. A wide range of normal ductal anatomic variants exist. The maximum size of the normal main pancreatic duct is 3 mm in adults and 5 mm in the elderly, which can be measured by computed tomography (CT) or ultrasound. The main pancreatic duct normally can be distended up to 7 mm during contrast injection for cholangiopancreatography. The pancreas develops without a capsule; this allows unrestricted extension of pancreatic secretions from a disrupted

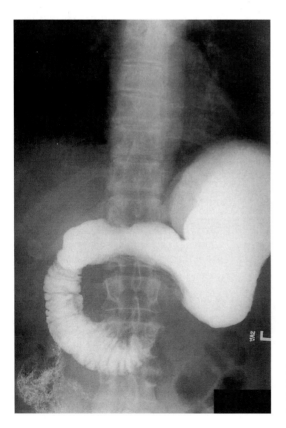

Figure 10–3. Pancreatic mass. Upper gastrointestinal series reveals a large pancreatic adenocarcinoma superiorly displacing the gastric antrum and deforming the duodenal C-loop.

gland into the adjacent tissues and unimpeded growth of pancreatic malignancies.

Imaging Modalities

Common indications for radiologic imaging of the pancreas include abdominal trauma, suspected pancreatitis, and suspected pancreatic neoplasm. Only gross pancreatic abnormalities can be suggested by conventional radiographs (Fig. 10–3). Magnetic resonance and angiography have limited roles in pancreatic imaging.

Computed tomography is the most commonly used imaging modality for evaluation of the pancreas (Fig. 10–4). Filling of adja-

cent bowel with water or other contrast agents as well as use of intravenous contrast is essential for optimal visualization. Without contrast, the borders of the pancreas can be difficult to discern because the gland is normally similar in attenuation to adjacent tissues. Optimal scanning is performed with narrow (routinely 5 mm) collimation, rapid bolus administration of intravenous contrast and rapid image acquisition times.

Ultrasonography of the pancreas can be difficult and is operator dependent (Fig. 10–5). Overlying bowel gas may obscure portions of the organ, but the left lobe of the liver can be used as an acoustic window. The stomach can be filled with water to serve as an additional sonographic window.

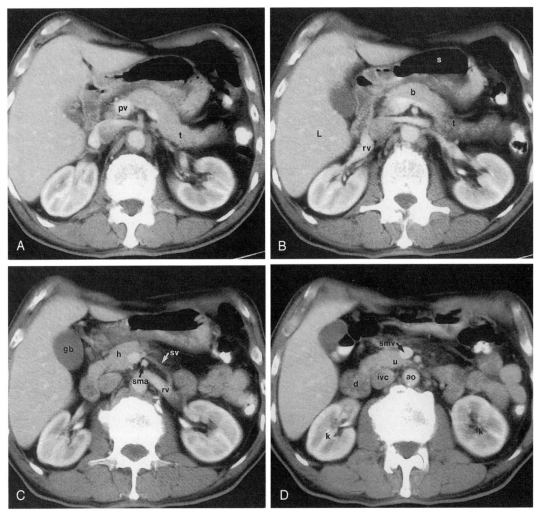

Figure 10–4. Normal CT scan of the pancreas. Contrast-enhanced axial CT images **(A through D)** illustrate the anatomic relationship of the normal pancreatic head (h), uncinate process (u), body (b), and tail (t) with adjacent structures: liver (L), stomach (s), duodenum (d), kidney (k), gallbladder (gb), aorta (ao), superior mesenteric artery (sma), inferior vena cava (ivc), portal vein (pv), renal veins (rv), and splenic vein (sv).

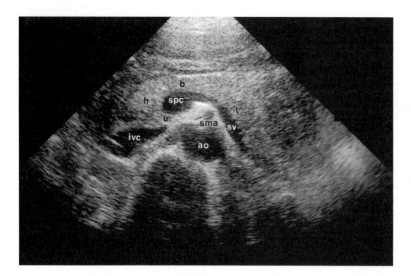

Figure 10–5. Normal ultrasound of the pancreas. Transverse sonogram demonstrates the pancreatic uncinate process (u), head (h), body (b), and tail (t). The splenic vein (sv) combines with the portal vein at the splenoportal confluence (spc). Echogenic fat surrounds the superior mesenteric artery (sma). The inferior vena cava (ivc) and aorta (ao) are visualized posteriorly.

Visualization of the pancreatic and bile ducts is achieved best with **endoscopic retrograde cholangiopancreatography (ERCP)**, in which the ductal system is cannulated endoscopically, injected with contrast and imaged fluoroscopically (Fig. 10–6). Calculi and iatrogenically introduced air bubbles create radiolucent intraluminal filling defects. Abnormal contours of the ducts may suggest pancreatic masses or chronic pancreatitis.

Structural Abnormalities

The pancreas develops from dorsal and ventral buds, which normally fuse during fetal development. Each bud has its own ductal system, and fusion between the ducts usually occurs, followed by partial regression of the dorsal duct. Failure of the buds to fuse causes **pancreas divisum,** in which two distinct pancreatic ductal segments persist (Fig. 10–7). Pancreas divisum is a relatively common congenital anomaly in which the uncinate process and pancreatic head are drained by the main pancreatic duct through the major papilla, and the remainder of the pancreas is drained by the accessory pancreatic duct through the minor papilla.

Fusion of a bifid ventral bud with the dorsal bud can result in **annular pancreas,** a rare condition in which a ringlike band of pancreatic tissue encircles the duodenum. Enlargement of this band of tissue, such as

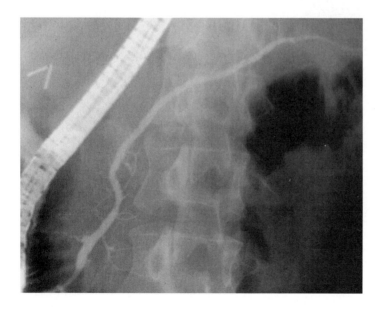

Figure 10–6. Normal ERCP. Endoscopic cannulation of the ampulla of Vater allows filling of the main pancreatic duct with iodinated contrast. The surgical clips in the right upper quadrant signify a prior cholecystectomy.

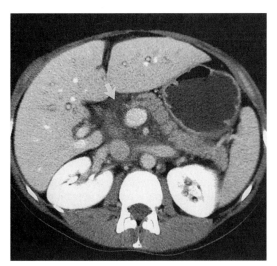

Figure 10–7. Pancreas divisum. Contrast-enhanced CT reveals two distinct pancreatic segments, separated by a cleft of fat *(arrow)*.

from inflammation or neoplastic growth, may result in duodenal obstruction. **Ectopic pancreatic tissue** is found in nearly 2% of the population, with common sites including the walls of the stomach and duodenum and in a Meckel diverticulum.

Fatty replacement of the pancreas is a common finding, especially in patients who are diabetic, obese, or elderly. **Pancreatic lipomatosis** and atrophy are associated with pancreatic insufficiency, but greater than 90% of the tissue must be nonfunctional to

result in clinical symptoms. The early manifestation of fatty replacement is an uneven marbled appearance on CT with lobules of fat interspersed among the pancreatic parenchyma; this creates a sonographically echogenic appearance. With advancing disease, the parenchyma can be obscured by fat, which blends into the retroperitoneal adipose tissue.

Congenital **cysts** of the pancreas are relatively uncommon and are thought to result from anomalous ductal development (Fig. 10–8). Pancreatic cysts are commonly seen in autosomal dominant polycystic disease and von Hippel–Lindau syndrome.

Acute Pancreatitis

Acute pancreatitis has a wide variety of causes, including infection, iatrogenic, mechanical, vascular, and metabolic causes (Table 10–1). Nearly 90% of cases are ac-

Table 10–1.
Causes of Acute Pancreatitis

Infectious
  Bacterial
  Viral (measles, mumps, HIV, CMV)
  Parasites (*Ascaris, Clonorchis*)
Iatrogenic
  Drugs (corticosteroids, diuretics, narcotics,
    estrogens)
  Postoperative
  Endoscopic retrograde cholangiopancreatography
Mechanical
  Cholelithiasis
  Trauma
  Pancreatic neoplasms
  Duodenal obstruction
  Choledochocele
Metabolic
  Alcohol
  Hyperlipidemia
  Kwashiorkor
  Diabetic ketoacidosis
  Uremia
  Hyperparathyroidism
Vascular
  Thrombosis
  Embolism
  Vasculitis (polyarteritis nodosa, SLE, Henoch-
    Schönlein purpura)
  Shock
Miscellaneous
  Pancreas divisum
  Hypothermia
  Pregnancy

CMV, cytomegalovirus; HIV, human immunodeficiency virus; SLE, systemic lupus erythematosus.

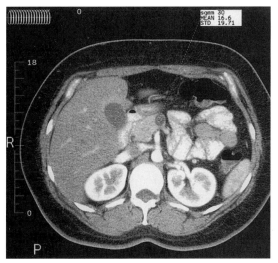

Figure 10–8. Congenital pancreatic cyst. A 2-cm low-attenuation lesion is present in the pancreatic body. Fluid content is confirmed as the cyst measures 16 HU, which is fluid attenuation.

counted for by alcoholism and biliary disease.

The common pathogenic process that unites the myriad varieties of acute pancreatitis is extravasation of pancreatic enzymes, which autodigest and ultimately necrose pancreatic and adjacent tissues. Pancreatic ductal obstruction can result from impacted gallstones, neoplasms, or inspissated proteinaceous plugs (seen in alcoholic pancreatitis). Acinar cell injury and deranged intracellular transport of enzymes are causative factors.

The diagnosis of pancreatitis is made clinically because imaging studies can be normal in mild cases. CT is the imaging modality of choice in pancreatitis and may show glandular edema, adjacent inflammatory changes,

necrosis, hemorrhage, abscess, or pseudocyst formation. Inflammation results in blurring of the organ contours, stranding of the peripancreatic fat, and thickening of surrounding fascial planes (Fig. 10–9).

Interstitial pancreatitis is the mildest form of the disease and is characterized by inflammation, which usually is accompanied by edema and minimal necrosis; this can result in a gland that is several times its normal size. Sonographically, there is reversal of the normal pattern of echogenicity, with the inflamed pancreas appearing hypoechoic to liver. Diagnosis by CT can be difficult in mild cases because the only manifestation may be subtle blurring of the peripancreatic fat (Fig. 10–10).

Necrotizing pancreatitis is a severe form

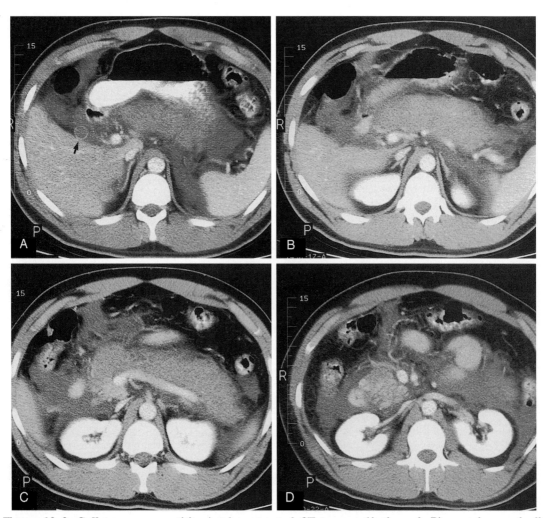

Figure 10–9. Gallstone pancreatitis. Axial contrasted CT images (**A** through **D**) reveal a markedly thickened pancreas with ill-defined borders and adjacent intraperitoneal fluid. A gallstone (*arrow* in **A**) is present in the gallbladder.

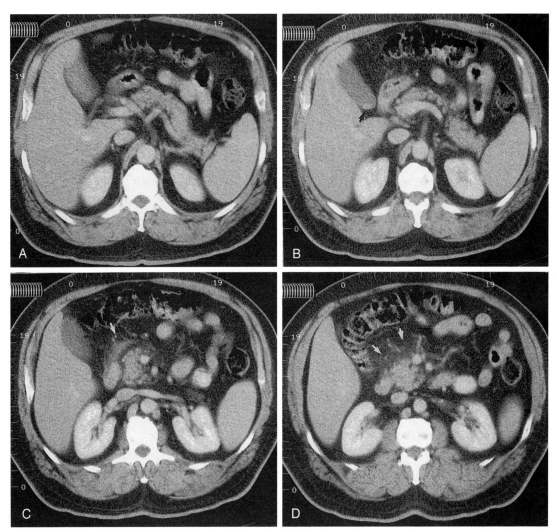

Figure 10–10. Interstitial pancreatitis. Axial contrasted CT images (**A** through **D**) illustrate how in mild cases of interstitial pancreatitis, the only manifestation may be faint blurring of the peripancreatic fat (*white arrows* in **C** and **D**). A radiopaque gallstone (*black arrow* in **B**) is present in the gallbladder.

of pancreatitis characterized by extensive fat necrosis, parenchymal hemorrhage, and necrosis of surrounding tissues. When hemorrhage predominates, it is termed ***hemorrhagic pancreatitis.*** Hemorrhage results from erosion of blood vessels and is seen as high-attenuation fluid in or adjacent to the pancreas. Vascular damage can result in **thrombosis,** especially involving the portal, splenic, and mesenteric veins.

A **pseudoaneurysm** can develop after arterial disruption with resulting encapsulation of hemorrhage. Pseudoaneurysms are extravascular hematomas that communicate with the intravascular space and differ from true aneurysms by lacking all three vascular tunics. Rupture of a pseudoaneurysm is gen-

erally fatal, making diagnosis imperative so that intervention, such as embolization of the feeding vessel, can be performed. Color Doppler ultrasound or contrast-enhanced CT can be used to distinguish a pancreatic pseudoaneurysm from a pseudocyst.

A **pseudocyst** is an encapsulated collection of pancreatic fluid that develops in the setting of inflammation, resulting from microperforation of the pancreatic ducts (Fig. 10–11). In contradistinction to **true cysts,** these structures lack a true epithelial lining. These lesions can be seen in acute and chronic pancreatitis and by definition must persist for at least 6 weeks. The lesions are commonly 5 to 10 cm in diameter, their walls range from thin and radiographically unde-

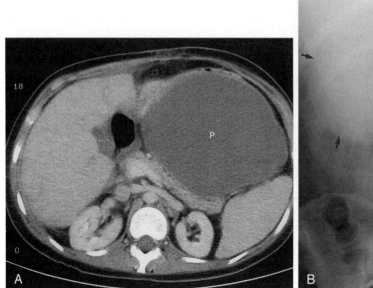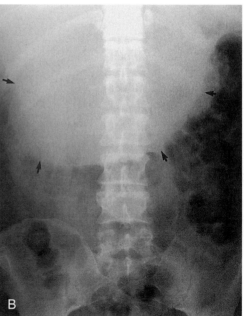

Figure 10–11. Pancreatic pseudocyst. A, A 16-cm pseudocyst (P) emanates from the body and tail of the pancreas, compressing the stomach and displacing it anteriorly. **B,** A conventional abdominal radiograph in another patient shows an elliptical area of soft tissue density *(arrows)*, representing a pseudocyst inferiorly displacing the transverse colon.

tectable to thick and fibrous, and they may contain calcium. Pseudocysts are commonly round or elliptical and are unilocular, which is helpful in differentiating from neoplastic cysts. Large pseudocysts occasionally can be seen on conventional radiographs. Nearly 50% of pseudocysts resolve spontaneously. The clinical significance of pseudocysts is related to size and potential complications because they can displace or compress adjacent structures, become infected, erode into adjacent vessels (Fig. 10–12), or rupture into the peritoneum resulting in **pancreatic ascites** or peritonitis. Because of these potential complications, pseudocysts greater than 5 cm are often drained internally or percutaneously.

Acute fluid collections, formerly termed *phlegmon,* are accumulations of pancreatic fluid that are seen in approximately 40% of patients with acute pancreatitis. These collections can have a similar appearance to pseudocysts but do not have a capsule. Ultimate differentiation depends on their life span, with half resolving spontaneously.

Fluid collections, necrosis, and hemorrhage provide a fertile environment for bacterial growth and formation of a **pancreatic abscess** (Fig. 10–13). Abscesses can be located in the gland parenchyma or in the peripancreatic tissues and often occur greater than 4 weeks after onset of acute pancreatitis. Abscesses can appear as ill-defined or loculated fluid collections and often are indistinguishable from uninfected fluid

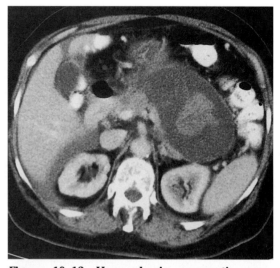

Figure 10–12. Hemorrhagic pancreatic pseudocyst. A large pseudocyst arises from the pancreatic body and tail and contains central high-attenuation material, representing contracted blood products from hemorrhage after vascular erosion.

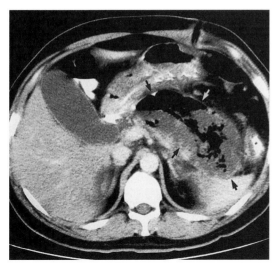

Figure 10–13. Pancreatic abscess. Gas collections are evident within a large pancreatic abscess *(arrows)*.

collections or pseudocysts. The presence of gas within the lesion from gas-forming bacteria is an infrequent (approximately 20%) but characteristic finding seen in abscesses. An enhancing rim of tissue may be seen on contrast-enhanced CT. Most abscesses are treated effectively by percutaneous drainage. Infected necrosis is a more severe complication that can appear at any time and usually necessitates surgical débridement.

Chronic Pancreatitis

Repeated bouts of inflammation with progressive destruction of pancreatic tissue, atrophy, impaired endocrine and exocrine function, and proliferation of fibrous tissue results in **chronic pancreatitis.** Hallmarks of chronic pancreatitis include parenchymal calcifications, intraductal calculi, fluid collections, fatty replacement, fibrosis, peripancreatic fat stranding, fascial thickening, and irregular dilation of the pancreatic duct (Fig. 10–14). Complications of chronic pancreatitis are similar to those of acute pancreatitis and can be seen on conventional radiographs, including calcifications and mass effect on adjacent structures.

Pancreatic Neoplasms

Pancreatic neoplasms can be divided into tumors of the exocrine pancreas, the endo-crine pancreas (islet cell neoplasms), and other tissue types. Virtually all pancreatic carcinomas originate from the ductal epithelium of the exocrine gland, with the acinar cells giving rise to less than 1% of pancreatic malignancies.

Exocrine neoplasms include adenocarcinoma, cystic neoplasms, and several rare tumors. **Endocrine neoplasms** arise from the amine precursor uptake and decarboxylation (APUD) system in the islets of Langerhans and include insulinomas, gastrinomas, VIPomas (producing vasoactive intestinal peptide), somatostatinomas, glucagonomas, and nonfunctioning islet cell tumors. Other pancreatic neoplasms include lymphoma, metastases, and mesenchymal tumors.

Adenocarcinoma is an extremely lethal malignancy that comprises 95% of all pancreatic tumors (Fig. 10–15). The 5-year survival rate is only 3%, and surgical resection offers the only chance of a cure. Resectability usually is assessed with contrast-enhanced CT. Approximately two thirds of adenocarcinomas arise in the pancreatic head, with about 5% being resectable. Involvement of the body and tail usually indicates unresectability. These neoplasms can result in ductal obstruction and can invade adjacent organs and blood vessels. Metastases to the liver are common, followed by regional lymph nodes, peritoneum, and lung.

Cystic pancreatic neoplasms mostly can be divided into two categories: microcystic adenoma and mucinous cystic neoplasms. **Cystic teratomas** occasionally arise in the pancreas and have the same imaging characteristics as seen in other parts of the body.

The benign **microcystic adenoma** (serous adenoma) is a hypervascular tumor that accounts for nearly half of the cystic pancreatic neoplasms. It is seen most commonly in elderly women and is composed of innumerable small cysts that coalesce into masses that average 13 cm in diameter. A classic finding, seen in 20% of cases, is a central stellate scar, which may calcify. These tumors show calcification more often than any other pancreatic neoplasm, and one third usually can be seen on conventional radiographs. On CT, this tumor has a characteristic "Swiss cheese" appearance.

Mucinous cystic neoplasms include the benign **mucinous cystadenoma** and the malignant **mucinous cystadenocarcinoma** (Fig. 10–16). These two tumors are difficult to distinguish radiographically and can be dif-

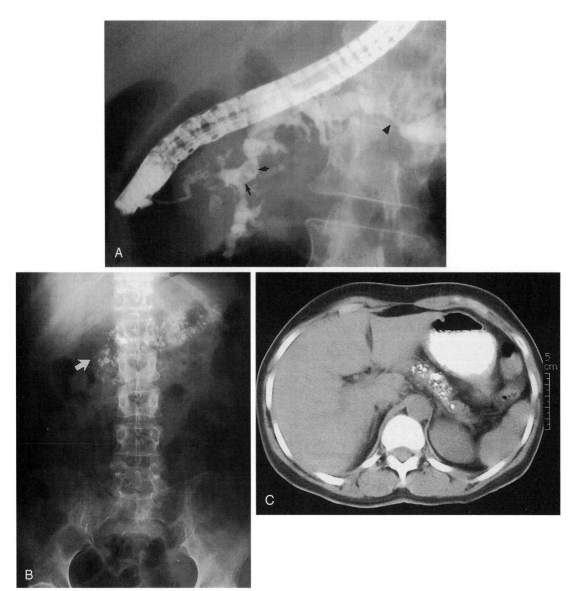

Figure 10–14. Chronic pancreatitis. A, A spot film from an ERCP shows irregular dilation of the main pancreatic duct with intraluminal filling defects resulting from multiple calculi *(arrows)*, as well as a stricture *(arrowhead)* of the distal duct. **B,** Conventional radiograph reveals multiple pancreatic calcifications *(arrow)*. **C,** Axial noncontrasted CT shows multifocal calcifications throughout the pancreatic parenchyma.

ferentiated reliably only histologically. They are hypovascular tumors that contain six or fewer cysts, which are each less than 20 mm in diameter.

Approximately 85% of **islet cell tumors** are functional, secreting one or more hormones. The most common functional islet cell neoplasm is the **insulinoma,** accounting for nearly 70% of these tumors. Insulinomas have a markedly low rate of malignancy, compared with the other islet cell tumors.

Numerous islet cell–type tumors have been described (Table 10–2). **Gastrinomas, VIPomas, somatostatinomas,** and **glucagonomas** are encountered less commonly. These hypervascular tumors generally are small and require optimal CT technique for visualization because they are generally isodense with normal pancreatic tissue on noncontrasted scans, but they enhance peripherally after bolus administration of intravenous contrast (Fig. 10–17). Functional

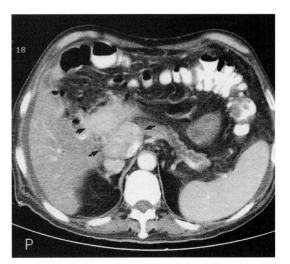

Figure 10–15. Pancreatic adenocarcinoma. A large soft tissue mass *(arrows)* originates from the head of the pancreas, a characteristic location for adenocarcinoma.

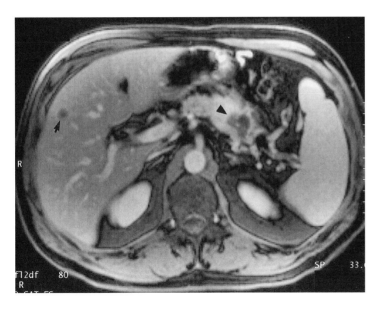

Figure 10–16. Mucinous cystadenocarcinoma. Axial T1-weighted postgadolinium MRI with fat saturation shows a hypointense mucinous cystadenocarcinoma of the pancreatic tail *(arrowhead)* with a liver metastasis *(arrow).*

Table 10–2.
Endocrine Pancreatic Neoplasms

Neoplasm	Cell of Origin	Hormone
Insulinoma	B	Insulin
Gastrinoma	G	Gastrin
VIPoma	Neuron	Vasoactive intestinal peptide
Somatostatinoma	D	Somatostatin
Glucagonoma	A	Glucagon
ACTHoma	?	Adrenocorticotropic hormone
Carcinoid	Enterochromaffin	Serotonin
Pancreatic polypeptidoma	PP	Pancreatic polypeptide
Nonfunctioning	?	None

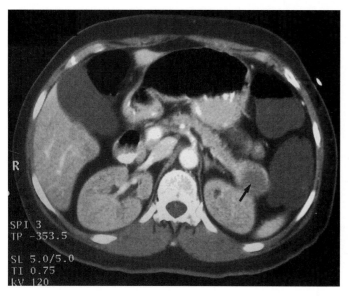

Figure 10–17. Pancreatic islet cell carcinoma. Axial contrasted CT reveals an expansile low-attenuation mass *(arrow)* in the tail of the pancreas. Accompanied by dilation of multiple loops of fluid-filled small bowel, this appearance is pathognomonic of Verner-Morrison syndrome, a rare condition of watery diarrhea, hypokalemia, and achlorhydria that is associated with high levels of vasoactive intestinal polypeptide resulting from a pancreatic VIPoma.

neoplasms can be benign or malignant, although there is a high rate of malignant transformation.

Nonfunctional islet cell tumors are characteristically larger than their functional counterparts and commonly range from 6 to 20 cm in size. This large size can be useful in differentiation from adenocarcinomas. Many tumors that are classified as nonfunctional actually secrete other substances, such as

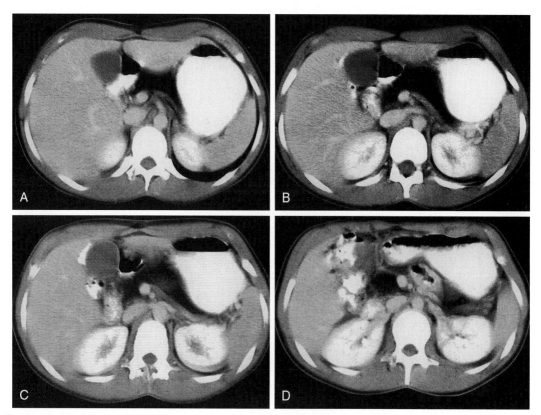

Figure 10–18. Cystic fibrosis. Sequential axial contrasted CT images (**A** through **D**) reveal no discernible pancreatic tissue, resulting from severe atrophy of the gland.

pancreatic polypeptide. Malignant transformation occurs in approximately 75% of nonfunctional islet cell neoplasms.

Miscellaneous Conditions

Pancreatic manifestations of **cystic fibrosis** result from viscous exocrine secretions that lead to progressive ectasia and obstruction of the pancreatic ductules with ensuing inflammation, atrophy, fibrosis, and fatty replacement (Fig. 10–18). Small (1 to 3 mm) cysts are common, but rarely are visualized radiographically.

Most pancreatic injuries are caused by penetrating trauma, such as gunshot and stab wounds. Because of the anatomic position of the pancreas between the anterior body wall and the spine, it is susceptible to injury in cases of blunt abdominal trauma, including motor vehicle accidents and child abuse. Pancreatic injuries include traumatic pancreatitis, contusion, laceration, and rarely transection. Although pancreatic injuries are relatively uncommon, they are associated with high morbidity and are correlated highly with concomitant visceral trauma. Because of the retroperitoneal location of the pancreas, injuries often are clinically occult.

Pancreatic **contusions** are most commonly isoattenuating on CT but as a result of intraparenchymal hemorrhage can be hyperattenuating. Contusions and hematomas can result in a focal area of bulging in the contour of the organ.

Lacerations are manifested by irregular clefts of low attenuation on CT, which may be intraparenchymal or extend to the surface. Lacerations are seen best after enhancement of the gland with intravenous contrast, which accentuates the cleft. Adjacent peripancreatic hemorrhage and blurring of fascial planes are signs of laceration.

Complete pancreatic **transection** (Fig. 10–19) is rare and is associated with nonenhancement of a segment of the gland because its arterial supply has been severed. Transection is a surgical emergency because it can lead to intraperitoneal hemorrhage

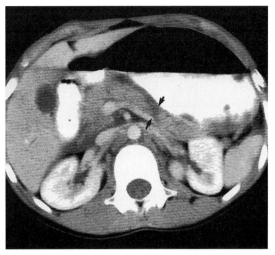

Figure 10–19. Traumatic pancreatic transection. Contrast-enhanced CT displays an irregular cleft *(arrows)* extending anteroposteriorly through the junction of the pancreatic body and tail with surrounding free intraperitoneal fluid in a 10-year-old girl after a motor vehicle accident.

and leakage of pancreatic enzymes with resultant destruction of adjacent tissues. Delayed complications of trauma include fistula, abscess, pancreatitis, and pseudocyst formation.

Pancreatic **transplantation** is a relatively uncommon procedure but can create a confusing radiographic picture. Transplantations can be segmental from a living donor or whole organ from a cadaveric donor. The transplant usually is positioned in the pelvis and anastomosed to the iliac vessels, although a variety of vascular anastomoses can be made. A favored strategy for diverting exocrine secretions is a duodenocystostomy.

Suggested Readings

Friedman AC, Dachman AH: Radiology of the Liver, Biliary Tract, and Pancreas. St. Louis, Mosby, 1994.

Gore RM, Levine MS, Laufer I: Textbook of Gastrointestinal Radiology, 2nd ed. Philadelphia, WB Saunders, 2000.

Webb WR, Brant WE, Helms CA: Fundamentals of Body CT, 2nd ed. Philadelphia, WB Saunders, 1998.

ELEVEN

Spleen

CECILIA M. COUTSIAS, M.D.

Normal Anatomy

The spleen, a part of the mononuclear-phagocytic system, is a markedly vascular intraperitoneal organ of the left upper quadrant; its functions include blood filtration by phagocytosis, antigen presentation, extramedullary hematopoiesis, and storage of cellular blood elements. Its vascularity has implications in the consequences of splenic trauma. Its filtering role puts it at risk for involvement in systemic diseases, such as infiltrative processes and metastatic malignancy.

The spleen is located posteriorly, lateral to the stomach and superior to the left kidney. Splenic morphology shows remarkable variety; it may be lenticular or crescentic and may display clefts, lobulations, and notches along its contours. Its variable shape poses a challenge to volumetric measurement, but in general, the longitudinal dimension of the spleen should not exceed 12 to 14 cm. On sonographic evaluation, the spleen should not extend beyond the inferior pole of the left kidney.

The parenchyma comprises alternating amorphous rests of red and white pulp, through which percolate the blood supplied by the **splenic artery,** a tortuous branch of the celiac axis. Blood is drained by the **splenic vein,** found immediately posterior to the pancreas, which then joins the superior mesenteric vein at the portal confluence (Fig. 11–1).

Imaging Modalities

Radiologic imaging of the spleen includes conventional radiographs (to a limited degree), ultrasonography, computed tomography (CT), magnetic resonance imaging (MRI), and nuclear medicine. **Conventional radiographs** of the abdomen may reveal the splenic contour outlined by intraperitoneal fat, but this is seen most commonly when the spleen is enlarged and displaces bowel from the left upper quadrant. Splenic and left lower lobe pulmonary granulomas project over the left upper quadrant and can be difficult to distinguish. The densely calcified autoinfarcted spleen of sickle cell anemia may be visible by conventional radiographs. Atherosclerotic calcification of the splenic artery may be apparent as curvilinear radiodensities situated to the left of the thoracolumbar junction.

Ultrasonography of the normal spleen reveals homogeneous parenchymal echotexture, usually isoechoic or slightly hyperechoic to liver. Doppler interrogation is useful in evaluation of splenic vein patency and in the assessment of reversal of flow in the case of portal venous hypertension. The

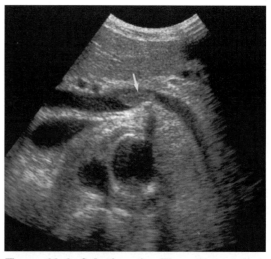

Figure 11–1. Splenic vein. The splenic vein is seen just posterior to the pancreas using ultrasonography. A small focus of intraluminal echogenicity *(arrow)* represents a thrombus at the junction of the splenic vein with the superior mesenteric vein at the portal confluence.

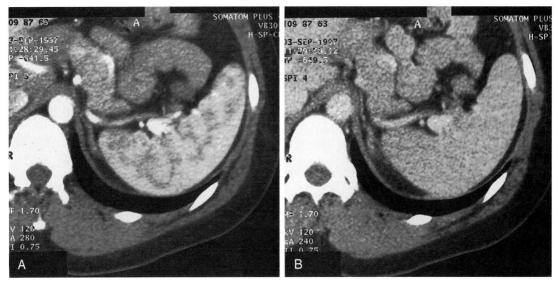

Figure 11–2. Moiré spleen. A, Early arterial phase contrasted CT demonstrates typical heterogeneous splenic enhancement caused by different flow rates through red and white pulp. **B,** Delayed imaging reveals homogeneous parenchymal attenuation.

spleen is employed commonly as an acoustic window for imaging of the left kidney.

On **CT,** the attenuation of the normal spleen is usually 8 to 10 HU less than the liver on precontrast and postcontrast imaging. With the advent of high-speed helical CT scanners, enabling imaging in early arterial phase, recognition of the heterogeneous **Moiré** or **wild spleen** early enhancement pattern prevents misclassification of a normal organ; delayed imaging should reveal homogeneous enhancement of the parenchyma (Fig. 11–2). CT is sensitive for, and of great utility in characterization of, splenic lesions.

The spleen typically shows long T1 and T2 relaxation times on **MRI.** T1 signal intensity generally is similar to renal cortex and slightly darker than hepatic parenchyma, whereas T2 signal of the spleen is normally brighter than liver. The ability to image in multiple planes makes MRI of particular utility in determining spatial relationship of the spleen with the left kidney, adrenal gland, and hemidiaphragm.

Nuclear medicine imaging depends on intravenously injected technetium 99m–labeled sulfur colloid or heat-damaged red blood cells that are sequestered by phagocytosis in the spleen; subsequent scintigraphic imaging yields information regarding the presence or absence of splenic tissue and splenic size as well as nonspecific information regarding filling defects implying the presence of a splenic mass.

Structural Abnormalities

Heterotaxy variants **asplenia** and **polysplenia** are associated with absent and multiple spleens, respectively. The presence or absence of splenic tissue can be assessed with certainty employing technetium 99m–labeled sulfur colloid or red blood cells or with angiography of the celiac axis (Fig. 11–3).

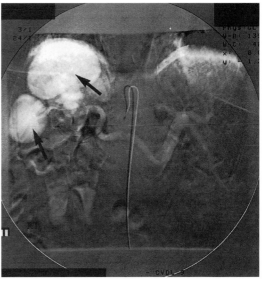

Figure 11–3. Polysplenia. Celiac arteriogram in a patient with situs inversus reveals multiple right-sided splenules *(arrows).*

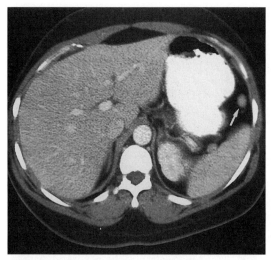

Figure 11–4. Accessory spleen. CT reveals a small, rounded structure just anterior to the spleen *(arrow)* that is of matching attenuation and compatible with a splenule.

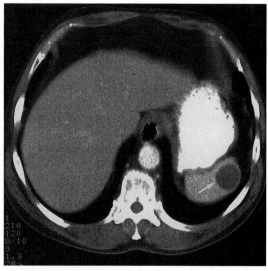

Figure 11–5. Epidermoid cyst. Contrasted CT illustrates a simple cystic structure *(arrow)* within the lateral aspect of the spleen, representing a small congenital cyst.

Small nodules of normal splenic tissue may form independently of the primary spleen; these **accessory (supernumerary) spleens** are typically found in the vicinity of the splenic hilum. They may be mistaken for adenopathy or pancreatic tail masses. Their true identity can be suggested by noting identical attenuation, signal intensity, or echogenicity with the main spleen (Fig. 11–4) and verified by the presence of radiopharmaceutical uptake in nuclear medicine sulfur colloid or heat-damaged red blood cell scans.

The spleen rarely may be tethered by a long, redundant and mobile mesentery, allowing its position within the abdomen to shift; this had been termed the ***wandering spleen.*** Occasionally the spleen may rotate about the long axis of this mesentery through which its vascular supply courses, leading to acute **torsion.** The patient presents with acute, and possibly intermittent, left upper quadrant pain. Doppler ultrasound may be of assistance in diagnosis.

Congenital splenic **cysts** typically are simple; termed ***epidermoid* cysts,** they are the only variety to contain an epithelial lining (Fig. 11–5). Pancreatic pseudocysts may extend into the spleen through the splenic hilum or may originate within the splenic parenchyma. A large splenic hematoma may not resolve completely, but gradually decrease in attenuation and echogenicity and develop a calcified rim (Fig. 11–6), resem-

bling a cyst. Echinococcal infection is manifested by single or multiple cystic structures, sometimes with a thinly calcified margin.

Splenomegaly may result from a multitude of pathologic processes and can be diagnosed with various imaging modalities (Fig. 11–7). Splenomegaly resulting from pas-

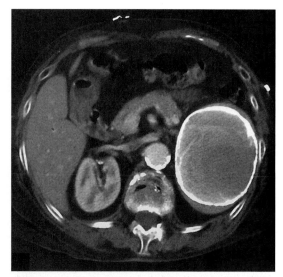

Figure 11–6. Remote splenic hematoma. Contrasted CT in a patient with remote history of trauma reveals dense calcification of the periphery of a complex fluid collection within the spleen, consistent with an old hematoma.

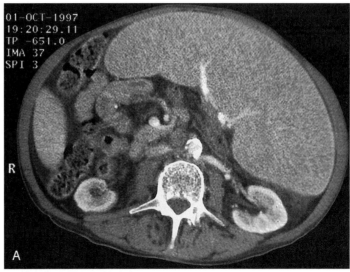

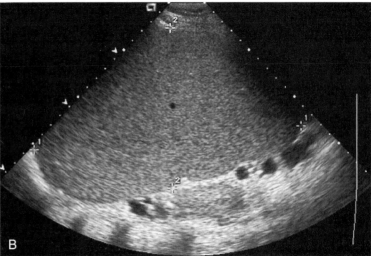

Figure 11–7. Splenomegaly. A, Contrasted CT at the level of the inferior hepatic tip reveals marked splenic enlargement in a patient with mantle cell lymphoma. **B,** Sonogram shows a markedly enlarged spleen (between calipers) in a 28-year-old woman with splenomegaly from portal hypertension. Portal venous hypertension was caused by cirrhosis that arose from primary sclerosing cholangitis.

sive congestion may be seen with right-sided heart failure and portal venous hypertension and may be accompanied by decreased attenuation or echogenicity of the swollen splenic parenchyma. Other causes include neoplastic infiltration (e.g., leukemia and lymphoma), infiltrative diseases (e.g., amyloidosis), storage diseases (e.g., Gaucher and Niemann-Pick), infectious processes (e.g., mononucleosis and malaria), and sarcoidosis.

Splenic Infection

Pyogenic abscesses of the spleen have a variable appearance but generally are low-attenuation, irregular lesions that may exhibit thickened, contrast-enhancing rinds;

they may contain gas bubbles (Fig. 11–8). Sonography reveals simple or complex fluid collections, with internal echoes, irregular walls, and enhanced through-transmission; the presence of gas may be reflected by "dirty" acoustic shadowing.

Prior **granulomatous disease** of the spleen leads to multiple punctate parenchymal calcifications easily seen by CT and ultrasound; etiologies most commonly include histoplasmosis and tuberculosis (Fig. 11–9). Sarcoidosis is a noninfectious cause of splenic granulomas.

Fungal infections of the spleen most commonly present as **microabscesses,** seen as small low-attenuation lesions on CT, and hypoechoic lesions on ultrasound. Such processes typically are seen in immunocompromised patients; common organisms

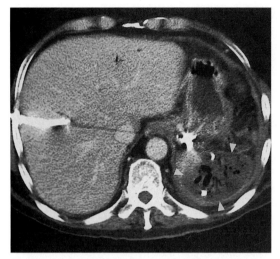

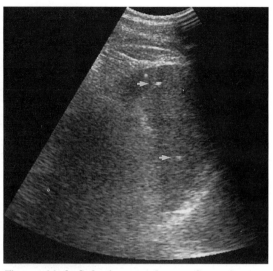

Figure 11–8. Splenic abscess. Contrasted CT in a patient with pancreatitis, who developed splenic infarction after repair of a splenic artery pseudoaneurysm, demonstrates progression of infarction to frank abscess *(arrowheads)*. The presence of a surgical drain within the fluid collection decreases the ability to suggest infection based on the presence of gas bubbles, as air can be introduced with catheter manipulation.

Figure 11–9. Splenic granulomas. Several punctate echogenic foci within the spleen *(arrows)* on sonographic evaluation are consistent with prior granulomatous disease. Small calcifications such as these may not cause acoustic shadowing.

include *Candida albicans* (Fig. 11–10), *Mycobacterium tuberculosis* (Fig. 11–11), and *Mycobacterium avium-intracellulare* (Fig. 11–12). The liver may be involved simultaneously (see Fig. 11–10). *Pneumocystis carinii* infec-

tion may lead to multiple focal calcifications within the spleen.

Benign Neoplasms

Tumors of the spleen are relatively uncommon and may show a variety of appear-

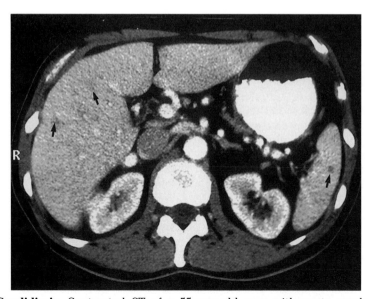

Figure 11–10. Candidiasis. Contrasted CT of a 55-year-old man with acute myelogenous leukemia displays subtle low-attenuation lesions *(arrows)* within the liver and the spleen, representing candidal microabscesses.

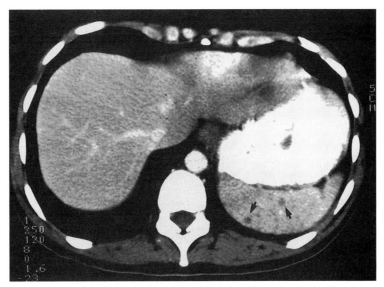

Figure 11–11. Tuberculosis. Contrasted CT in patient with disseminated *Mycobacterium tuberculosis* infection reveals multiple small, rounded, low-attenuation microabscesses *(arrows)* within the spleen.

ances. Benign neoplasms include **lymphangioma,** which most commonly presents as a multicystic mass containing simple fluid on ultrasound and CT. **Hemangiomas** may display a variety of appearances; they may be hyperechoic by sonography, similar to those seen in the liver. Hemangiomas may contain phleboliths. On contrast-enhanced CT, they may show early peripheral nodular contrast enhancement with gradual central filling on delayed images, also reminiscent of hepatic findings (Fig. 11–13).

Malignant Neoplasms

Malignancy of the spleen includes such primary tumors as **hemangiosarcoma** and **angiosarcoma** (the latter associated with Thorotrast administration in the 1950s).

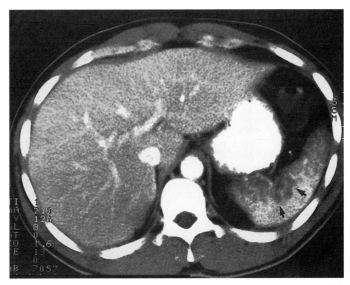

Figure 11–12. *Mycobacterium avium-intracellulare* infection. Contrasted CT of 36-year-old man with acquired immunodeficiency syndrome illustrates multiple small, rounded hypoattenuating lesions *(arrows)* within the spleen, some of which are confluent, representing opportunistic *M. avium-intracellulare* infection.

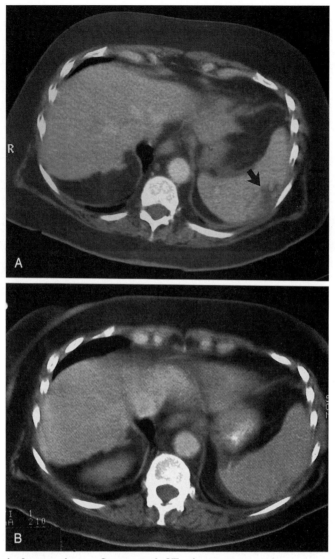

Figure 11–13. Splenic hemangioma. Contrasted CT of a patient with an irregular hypoattenuating splenic lesion *(arrow)* demonstrates discontinuous early peripheral enhancement **(A),** with central filling on later images **(B);** this is classic for hemangioma, which is seen more commonly in the liver.

AIDS-related lymphoma and **Kaposi sarcoma** are manifested by single or multiple solid lesions. **Lymphoma** and **leukemia** may involve the spleen; they may reveal diffuse splenic infiltration and enlargement or single or multiple low-attenuation and hypoechoic lesions (Fig. 11–14). A granulomatous disease rather than a neoplasm, such as **sarcoidosis,** also may manifest as multiple low-attenuation splenic lesions (Fig. 11–15).

Metastases are most commonly from malignant melanoma, but also include adenocarcinoma of ovary, breast, lung, and stomach (Fig. 11–16). Metastases may be solid or cystic in nature and may be multiple or solitary.

Miscellaneous Conditions

The spleen is the intraperitoneal solid organ most vulnerable to injury from **trauma.** CT is the most sensitive and timely modality in evaluation, although sonographic evaluation of the noncritical patient in the emergency department may play a role. Contained parenchymal **hematoma** is seen as an irregular low-attenuation or hypoechoic

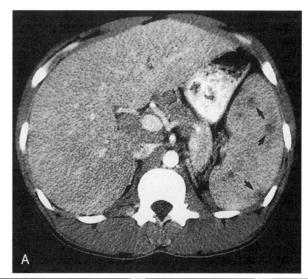

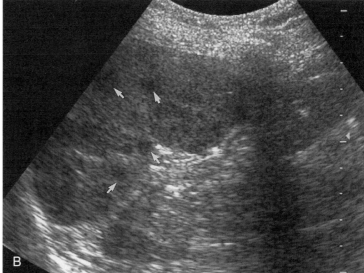

Figure 11–14. Lymphoma. A, Contrasted CT of a 29-year-old man with acquired immunodeficiency syndrome with Hodgkin lymphoma reveals multiple subtle low-attenuation splenic lesions *(arrows)* and porta hepatis and periaortic adenopathy. **B,** Splenic sonogram reveals several faintly hypoechoic lesions *(arrows)* from lymphomatous involvement of non-Hodgkin lymphoma. **C,** Contrasted CT of a 25-year-old man shows several hypoattenuating lesions *(arrows)* within the spleen, one leading to anterior bulging of the splenic contour and possible gastric invasion, from lymphomatous involvement.

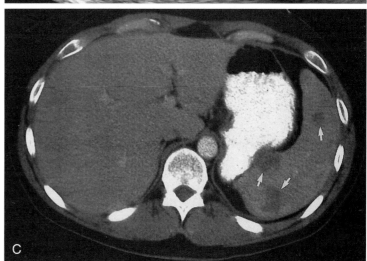

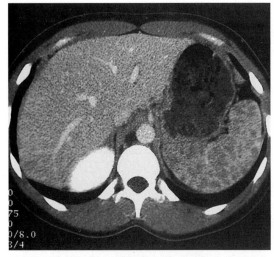

Figure 11–15. Sarcoidosis. CT displays multiple tiny low-attenuation splenic lesions *(arrows)* in a black woman with known sarcoidosis.

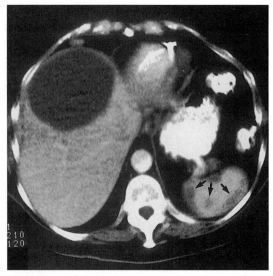

Figure 11–16. Splenic metastasis. Contrasted CT of a woman with hepatic biliary cystadenocarcinoma demonstrates multiple low-attenuation splenic lesions *(arrows)*, representing metastatic deposits.

focus. A crescentic low-attenuation fluid collection following the peripheral margin of the spleen is consistent with a **subcapsular hematoma;** this may be seen to distort the parenchymal contour if large enough to exert mass effect.

A **splenic laceration** is seen as a low-attenuation linear structure traversing the spleen and commonly extending to the capsule, in which case there may be associated perisplenic hemorrhage or frank hemoperito-

neum (Fig. 11–17). Hyperacute blood displays a higher attenuation on CT than does subacute blood. A **splenic cleft** may mimic a laceration; careful evaluation of contiguous slices should reveal the true nature of this anatomic variant (Fig. 11–18).

Splenic rupture may be life-threatening if associated with massive intraperitoneal

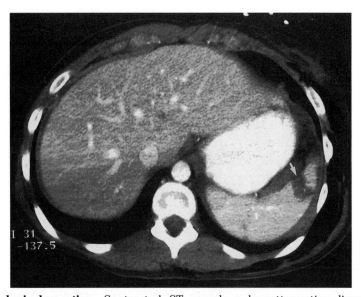

Figure 11–17. Splenic laceration. Contrasted CT reveals a low-attenuation linear defect *(arrow)* through the lateral aspect of the spleen, consistent with laceration, with small associated perisplenic hemorrhage and a small contusion posteromedially in a motor vehicle accident victim.

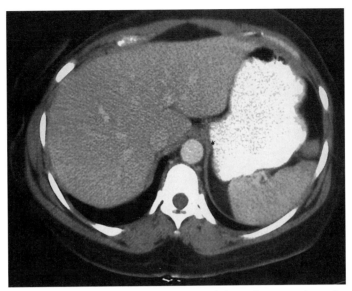

Figure 11–18. Splenic cleft. CT reveals a normal variant cleft at the anterolateral aspect of the spleen, which mimics a laceration in this patient without history of trauma.

hemorrhage; rapid diagnosis is essential (Fig. 11–19). Rupture of the spleen may be delayed temporally relative to the traumatic event, and reimaging with CT may be necessary if the patient's clinical status worsens, with dropping of the hematocrit. Complete disruption of the vascular pedicle may lead to absence of any normal parenchymal enhancement.

Whether managed by splenectomy or conservatively, if the rupture is relatively contained, seeding of the peritoneal cavity with splenic tissue may lead to the presence of multiple scattered small splenules, termed *splenosis.* These splenules may be found within the pelvis and, in cases of diaphragmatic breach, the pleural space. Diagnosis is confirmed with nuclear medicine sulfur colloid or heat-damaged red blood cell scans.

Splenic artery aneurysms are uncommon and typically have eggshell calcification (Fig. 11–20). They are more common in women with medial dysplasia of the wall. Pregnant women with a splenic artery aneurysm have a particularly increased risk of rupture of the aneurysm. Atherosclerosis is the major cause of splenic artery aneurysms in men.

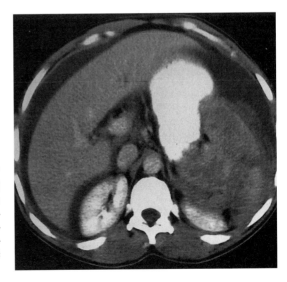

Figure 11–19. Splenic rupture. Contrasted CT shows a markedly fragmented spleen, with foci of low-attenuation hematoma centrally in a man struck with a baseball bat. Low-attenuation intraperitoneal fluid is consistent with hemoperitoneum; higher attenuation fluid immediately adjacent to the spleen suggests more acute hemorrhage.

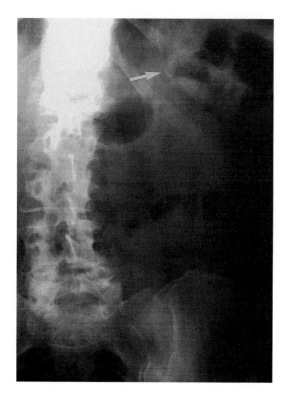

Figure 11–20. Splenic artery aneurysm. Abdominal radiograph reveals a rounded calcification in the left upper quadrant *(arrow)* representing a splenic aneurysm.

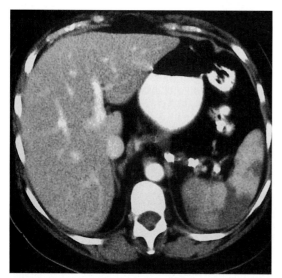

Figure 11–21. Splenic infarction. CT demonstrates several low-attenuation, peripherally based splenic lesions that are consistent with infarcts after splenic artery aneurysm embolization. Multiple embolization coils are seen within the splenic artery.

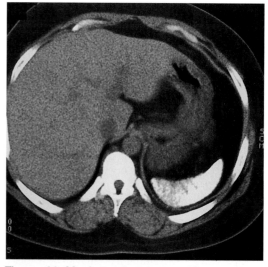

Figure 11–22. Autosplenectomy. Noncontrasted CT in a 27-year-old woman with sickle cell anemia reveals a small, densely calcified spleen.

Splenic infarction most commonly occurs subsequent to embolic events, usually of cardiac origin, such as from atrial fibrillation with left atrial thrombus or from bacterial endocarditis; other organs such as the kidneys may reveal infarcts. Less frequently, direct compression of splenic arterial supply by adjacent tumor or lymphadenopathy may be the cause. As with other organs, splenic infarcts typically are wedge-shaped, peripherally based lesions, showing low attenuation on contrasted CT (Fig. 11–21). Sonography reveals hypoechoic lesions acutely, which gradually become hyperechoic as fibrosis develops over time. Multiple infarcts may coalesce into irregular shapes, no longer conforming to the typical wedge-shaped description. Sickle cell anemia frequently leads to **autosplenectomy,** with small, densely calcified splenic remnant visible by multiple modalities (Fig. 11–22).

Suggested Readings

Dachman AH, Friedman AC: Radiology of the Spleen. St. Louis, Mosby Year-Book, 1993.

Friedman AC, Dachman AH: Radiology of the Liver, Biliary Tract, Pancreas, and Spleen, 2nd ed. St. Louis, Mosby-Year Book, 1994.

Haaga JR, Lanzieri CF, Sartoris DJ, Zerhouni EA: Computed Tomography and Magnetic Resonance of the Whole Body, 3rd ed. St. Louis, Mosby-Year Book, 1994.

Lee JK, Sagel SS, Stanley RJ, Heiken JP: Computed Body Tomography with MRI Correlation, 3rd ed. Philadelphia, Lippincott-Raven, 1998.

Webb WR, Brant WE, Helms CA: Fundamentals of Body CT, 2nd ed. Philadelphia, WB Saunders, 1991.

Index